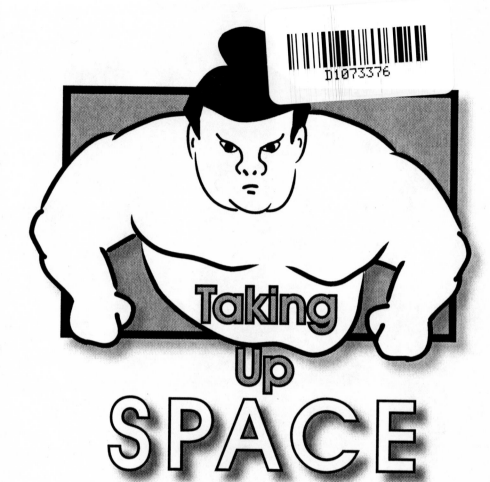

Taking Up SPACE

How Eating Well & Exercising Regularly Changed My Life

Pattie Thomas, Ph.D.

with *Carl Wilkerson, M.B.A.*

foreword by *Paul Campos*

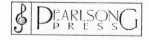
PEARLSONG PRESS

D1073376

Pearlsong Press
P.O. Box 58065
Nashville, TN 37205
www.pearlsong.com
1-866-4-A-PEARL

ISBN-13: 978-1-59719-002-2
ISBN-10: 1-59719-002-0
Library of Congress Control Number: 2005907296

Original trade paperback

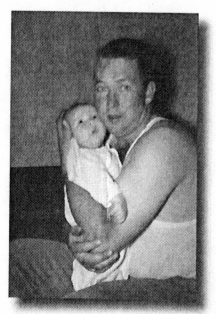

Photo 1957 LaVelle Thomas

This book is dedicated to my father,
Rufus Ray Thomas
(1929-1999).

His philosophy that American society
went downhill when people stopped
building front porches on houses
is the single greatest influence
on my becoming a sociologist.

I write this book in the hope
that we can soon start
being more neighborly.

See you on the front stoop.

Contents

Illustrations

Photos

Drawings

Foreword

For the last several years the media have helped
fuel our national hysteria about weight through their uncritical
acceptance of the government's definition of "overweight." A study
published in the April 23, 2005 issue of the *Journal of the American
Medical Association (JAMA)* may help lessen this hysteria, by turning
the widely accepted definition of "healthy weight" on its head.

According to our public health agencies, a healthy weight requires
a body mass index (BMI) between 18.5 and 24.9. People with a BMI
above 25 are "overweight;" those above 30 are "obese." The story we're
typically fed by the government and the media is that "overweight"
increases health risk significantly, while "obesity" is a deadly disease.
The new *JAMA* study conveys with special force just how wrongheaded
these definitions are.

Lead author Katherine Flegal of the Centers for Disease Control
(CDC) and the University of California-Berkeley analyzed data from
three representative samples of more than 36,000 Americans, covering
the years 1971 through 1994. Flegal and her colleagues asked the following question: After controlling for age, sex, race, smoking status,
and alcohol consumption, what sort of associations remain between
weight and mortality?

The answers will shock anyone who has relied on our government for information regarding the risks of being so-called "overweight."

Consider five women: Ann, Ellen, Lisa, Sarah, and Zoe. All are of average height (5'4"), but each has a different body type. Ann, who is fashionably thin, weighs 100 pounds. Ellen, who maintains what our public health authorities consider an ideal body mass, weighs 120 pounds. Lisa weighs 155 pounds, and is therefore "overweight" according to government standards. By these standards Sarah (185 pounds) and Zoe (240 pounds) are obese and severely obese, respectively. How do the *JAMA* study's findings apply to people at these different weight levels?

The study found that "obesity" was associated with approximately 112,000 excess deaths in the year 2000. This sounds like a large number, but in fact it represents a nearly four-fold reduction from the estimate made by a similar CDC study published spring 2004—a study that was subjected to such withering methodological criticism that the CDC took the extraordinary step of partially retracting its conclusions.

But this is the least startling of the authors' findings. The 112,000 excess deaths estimate was produced by comparing the mortality rates of supposedly "ideal weight" people (like Ellen) to those of "obese" people (like Sarah and Zoe). But when they compared the mortality rates of people like Ellen to those of people such as Lisa (i.e., the "overweight"), the authors uncovered a stunning result: the "ideal weight" group suffered 86,000 excess deaths in comparison to the "overweight" group!

In other words, in the year 2000, nearly as many excess deaths were associated with the government's "healthy" weight range as were associated with so-called "obesity." Meanwhile, "underweight" people (like Ann) endured a death rate far higher than that seen among the so-called "obese."

When you add up the numbers, it turns out the study found *fewer* excess deaths among Americans who weighed more than the government's recommended maximum than among those who weighed less, even though people in the former category outnumbered those in the latter.

Two points in particular stand out from the Flegal study's data: First, almost all excess risk associated with body mass is found in two groups: the underweight, and the extremely fat.

Second, the government's definition of "overweight"—the category that includes most Americans said to weigh too much—is completely bogus. The authors' data on this point is overwhelming: In all three of their subject groups, spanning nearly a quarter century, the so-called "overweight" faced a lower risk of premature death than did people of supposedly ideal weight.

In short, the diet doctors who have hijacked public health policy by getting the 75 million Americans with the lowest mortality risk classified as "overweight" have pulled off one of the most profitable scams in the history of junk science.

Although all this contradicts the conventional wisdom that feeds the current panic over fat, there is nothing particularly new about the authors' findings. Literally hundreds of medical studies suggest precisely what Flegal and her colleagues have demonstrated with such statistical force.

Indeed, if our public health authorities continue to cling to their absurd beliefs regarding the relationship between weight and health, while adjusting their definitions to the relevant data, they ought to recommend that Ellen gain 35 pounds so she can join Lisa in their new "ideal weight" category.

Luckily, there is no need to mimic the perverse logic of the war on fat by declaring an equally ridiculous war on thinness. **We need to recognize that weight is a cosmetic, cultural and political issue, not a medical one.** The sooner we acknowledge this, the sooner we will stop classifying perfectly healthy people as diseased, while at the same time worshiping a level of thinness that actually does correlate with greatly increased health risk. Once this is recognized, the health of women like Ann, Ellen, Lisa, Sarah, and Zoe, and the health of men with similar diversity in body size, will be improved.

What fuels America's irrational hatred of body diversity?

Overestimating a risk factor by 1,600% is a fairly spectacular mistake. Still, in reporting on the Flegal study's findings the media missed the real scandal: how a malignant combination of junk science, lazy journalism, and cultural prejudice has produced one of the longest and most destructive moral panics in American history.

First, the junk science: The supposedly shocking conclusion of the new study—that "overweight" people face a lower mortality risk than "ideal weight" individuals—was, in fact, unsurprising to objective observers who've studied the medical literature.

As anyone who is familiar with the evidence and isn't being paid to believe otherwise will attest, medical science has never supported the idea that so-called "overweight" people (people with a body mass index between 25 and 30) have a lower life expectancy or worse overall health than so-called "normal" or "ideal-weight" persons.

Indeed quite often, as in this new study, such "overweight" persons have the *highest* life expectancy within the studied population. And while it's true that the "overweight" are at a higher risk for certain diseases, such as diabetes and hypertension, the "ideal weight" among us are at higher risk for others, such as lung cancer and osteoporosis.

In short, this new study merely helps confirm what should already have been obvious: that the "overweight" category—the category that includes most Americans who the government claims weigh too much—is completely phony.

How did a scientifically bankrupt definition become the basis for the claim that two-thirds of us are dangerously fat? That's a complex story, but here is one piece of it.

Over the past decade an enormous amount of money, institutional power, and media attention has been dedicated to the claim that being "overweight"—not "obese," note, but merely "overweight"—is, in the words of Harvard Medical School Professor Walter Willett, "a major contributor to morbidity and mortality."

As I've documented at length elsewhere, this claim is simply bizarre. It is, I repeat, completely unsupported by the medical evidence. It's the equivalent of claiming that marijuana ought to be categorized as a Schedule I drug—that is, a highly dangerous drug that has no known medical use.

But of course marijuana *is* classified as a Schedule I drug, because the government's classification of marijuana has nothing to do with science, and everything to do with politics. The claim that 75 million Americans are "overweight," even though they face no increased overall health risk and indeed have a higher life expectancy than their supposedly ideally slim peers, is a product of similar factors. It is completely irrational. (By contrast, the claim that obesity is a major health risk is perhaps only about 97% false.)

Journalists believe this claim for all sorts of reasons. They believe it because it's much easier to quote the same people that are always quoted on an issue than it is to do any actual reporting. And they believe it because it usually reflects their own prejudices on this particular subject.

Most of all they believe it for the same reason so many obesity researchers believe it—because in a nation that spends $50 billion per year searching for non-existent weapons of body mass destruction, it pays to do so. Over the past couple of years I've interviewed several academics who told me they started featuring the supposed "obesity crisis" in grant applications because it was the easiest way to get funded. Those same funding sources are spending vast amounts of advertising dollars, including sponsoring news media and other journalism outlets. This $50 billion per year fuels the diet-pharmaceutical industrial complex—and, like the military-industrial complex of the Cold War, it will take a lot to break these financial interests.

Claiming that higher than average weight is a major health risk is extremely profitable, and, in a culture that loathes body fat, extremely plausible. It is, in other words, exactly the sort of claim that competent journalists should treat with skepticism.

The real scandal of the *JAMA* study is that it came as a bombshell. The study was a bombshell to the American media for one reason: because, in regard to this subject, they've failed to do their job.

Fortunately, there are signs that the current irrational panic over fat is giving birth to backlash among doctors, scientists, eating disorder specialists, sociologists, political scientists, and other scholars who have examined the evidence for the claims put forth by our fat-hating medical and public health establishments, and have discovered how slim or non-existent that evidence truly is.

Taking Up Space is an important contribution to this growing literature. Pattie Thomas is a sociologist by training, and her academic background is evident in the keen analytical eye she brings to bear on the question of just how and why fat has come to be demonized in our culture. But just as important, she uses the material of her own life experience to enrich that analysis with the insights gained by someone who spent much of her life at war with her own body, trying to conform to the crazy messages with which fat people in America are constantly bombarded.

In the course of doing so, she reveals how complex questions such as "what is health?" truly are, especially in regard to the much-misunderstood concept of "healthy weight." The powerful story of her own struggle with these issues highlights how absurd and destructive it is to label the heavier than average as diseased. That story also casts light on the depredations of the weight loss industry, which preys on fat people by selling them useless, expensive, and dangerous products that cause all sorts of health problems that, perversely enough, are then attributed to fat.

Taking Up Space is both a powerful work of scholarship and an inspiring personal account of what it means to be fat in America today. Readers of this book will come away with a renewed sense of how crucial it is to fight the moral panic that has enveloped us regarding this issue, and with a deep sense of admiration for people such as Pattie Thomas, and her co-author and partner Carl Wilkerson, who are on the front lines of this battle every day.

Paul Campos
University of Colorado School of Law
Author, *The Diet Myth*
(originally published as *The Obesity Myth)*
May 2005

Pattie's Preface

We have set down in the following pages what some might call a sociological memoir. It is a story of my life. But it is a story told in a greater context, and it is, therefore, more than a memoir. It is an analysis of my story in light of that greater context.

It is my hope that those who read this memoir can see themselves and their lives reflected in my story. It is also my hope that those who read this analysis can learn more about how to examine and analyze their own lives within their own social contexts. In essence, we are presenting a case study as much as we are presenting a narrative.

I am aware that my story has social and political implications, but I did not tell my story because I wanted to effect social change or because I wanted to be political. I have told this story because the storytelling itself was important to my personal development. I have told this story because I wanted to make sense of my own life. I have told this story because as a sociologist, I wanted to understand the context of my life.

I was not the one who made my body and my life politically charged or socially unjust. I hesitated to tell this story because I really don't want to be a "professional" fat person or a "professional" disabled person. But I am fat, and I am disabled. I cannot ignore these facts. They are central to many of my relationships with other people.

15

They are central to my own struggles and opportunities for personal development.

All of my goals for telling this story could have been accomplished through a personal diary, and, in fact, much of what is written in this book started out as either personal diary entries or as entries in my weblog. But I chose to write my story in the form of a book, and to find a publisher for that book, because I believed that not only will the content of my discoveries be important to other people—especially other stigmatized people—but also that the process I employed will be useful to anyone who takes the time to read this book.

So as you read my story, I invite you to see the process as well as the content. My process is marked by, although not limited to, five precepts:

1. *What other people choose to do counts.* Feeling good about myself was not enough to change how the world treated me. The choices other people make have an effect on my life, and I needed to develop responses to their choices that asserted my worth.

    I know that there are many gurus out there who believe that all you need is a positive attitude and everything will be okay. I believe in personal choice as well, but ignoring the effect of other peoples' choices is a poor strategy. I needed to react as well as I acted. That meant that I needed a strong understanding of the mechanisms that affected my life through the attitudes and actions of others.

2. *The social world works to our advantage as well.* I checked out my thinking by working with other people. Carl Wilkerson was central to this part of my process. Every idea I developed in this book and every part of my written story was created in conjunction with Carl. He and I spent a great deal of time talking out specific passages to make sure I was saying what I meant and meaning what I said.

    Everyone needs a sounding board in order to clarify one's thinking and feelings. A number of other people besides Carl were a part of my storytelling. I didn't always do what others asked of me, but I listened when they were willing to talk and I asked myself important questions in light of what they said.

I believe that people are basically social in nature. That means that I needed more than myself to develop and grow.

3. *Be patient. Growth takes time.* The nature of life is change. I am fond of saying that we tell many stories about our lives, and those stories change over time and never remain consistent. This is the story that I am telling about my life at this time. Actually, even this book has changed over time, as my story has changed while I have been writing the book.

This was a good time for me to write this story, because I feel somewhat satisfied with who I am and where I am going. I feel like I've worked out some big chunks of understanding my life and the context of my life. So now is a good time to share. There may be other stories to tell at other times.

4. *Skepticism is an important standpoint when examining the world and self.* We know, or at least strongly suspect, many things, without really thinking about how we know them. Asking the question about how I know what I know is tracing my knowledge back to its origins. Did I hear that on television? Did I think about something that led me to that conclusion? Did I read about this?

It doesn't really matter *where* I learned something for the purposes of the specific question, or whether it would be considered true or valid by some external standard. What matters is that *I know where I learned it.* If I don't know how I know what I know, then there is a good chance that I picked it up as simply a *given.* That would make it either a *habit* or an unexamined *norm.*

Habits and norms are important for human interaction. Without them, we would have to reinvent the wheel every time we had a conversation with other people. Knowing what to expect from others (norms) and reacting to those expectations without having to think about those reactions (habits) ensures everyday interactions run smoothly.

But when we rely too heavily upon habits and norms, we run the risk of repeating junk knowledge and reinforcing that knowledge in our culture. We run the risk of making something that is harmful feel natural. To guard against this, we need to question how we know what we know.

So if I can't answer the question "How do I know what I know?" then I know it is time to give some thought to that piece of information—some skeptical and critical thought. This is how we learn about the influence others have on our thinking, our beliefs, our attitudes, and our world views. This is where growth can occur. To ask critical questions is to better understand what you know and how you know. To ask critical questions will make you a stronger person.

5. *Criticizing something is not the same as hating it.* Upon reading this book many may come to the conclusion that I have no love for corporations. I am highly critical of the current health, beauty, diet, and fitness industries. I am highly suspicious of an economy based upon consumption for the sake of consumption. However, I consider the marketplace to be an exciting place. I like the creative energy that new enterprises engender. I like the interpersonal exchange of making transactions. I consider commerce a primary method of social interaction in our society.

When we exchange things, buy things, sell things, advertise things, and throw away things, we create culture in the sense that we create a basis for *shared meaning* in our social exchanges. Those shared meanings shapes the lives we live and limits the choices we have. That is why it is important when understanding stigma and the creation of stigma to understand the part commerce plays in that creation.

The critiques in this book are critiques of industries that have decided that conformity and social control are good business. This path leads to waste of human resources, because the contributions of so many worthwhile people are discounted on an arbitrary basis, and waste of physical resources because so much energy and effort is put into propositions and schemes that never improve lives or expand knowledge.

So as you read my assessments of the health, beauty, diet, and fitness industries, I invite you to consider that there may be other ways of doing commerce in these industries. Do not frame this discussion in the worn-out categories of "pro-business" and "anti-business." More choices are available to us to improve commerce. That is why I think critically about commerce. Far from being anti-capitalist, I believe in truly free capitalism, and I hope this book contributes to freer modes of commerce.

Yes, this story is about fat acceptance. Yes, this story is about the social stigma placed upon people. Would I like for you to examine your attitudes and beliefs about fatness, disability, and stigma by reading my story? Of course. But I hope for more for you as a reader.

What is outlined in this book is a story of growth and development examined in the social context of stigma. I invite you to read it as such. I invite you to examine your own life within that process. If you find that my processes help you create your own processes, I will feel rewarded for sharing this story.

If you'd like to share your stories with me, please drop me an e-mail at **drpattiethomas@threewisetwins.com**.

Cheers,
Pattie
March 2005

Carl's Preface

It took a lot to turn a 300-pound woman into the love of my life. But in one sense, it didn't take much more than it would have for any other woman.

I met Pattie Thomas when she was 5'1" tall and around 165 pounds. She was already over the so-called "normal" BMI, as you can probably guess without having to look up the specific values in a table thereof. But she was smart, seductive, and capable of carrying on a conversation without having to take breaks every five minutes to rest her brain. We were engaged within six months of meeting. We married a year after that.

Pattie never seemed as obsessed with her weight as other people were. She dieted, and she read up on nutrition, but she always seemed to consider it only one aspect of her life. Given her various other gifts and experiences, her perspective on the matter was, to my perception, reasonable.

I was never entirely pleased with Pattie's weight. However, like her, I was at least perceptive enough to note that there was more to her than her measurements. In fact, we did a thorough enough job of hacking through our relationship issues that by August of 1995 (about three years after being wed), I realized and related to her that the only thing that I found really troublesome about her was her size.

She wasn't pleased with the remark (which I had meant more to indicate how well things were going overall) and let me know so. She needn't have bothered pursuing the point at all: I was about to get an extensive internship whose theme was to be just how insignificant a thing like girth could become in the life of an adult couple.

Pattie and I were forced to live apart for three months in 1995. She had been admitted to a graduate program at Boston College, and I remained in Florida while she attended classes that autumn. We planned to remain apart for the duration of her studies, with exceptional visits during long breaks in her classes. After about a month of physical separation, our wills broke, and our telephone bills and e-mail inboxes became so crammed with line items that we realized we could get along a lot better *with* each other than without each other. I was reminded of the joke about two men conversing on the street. One asks after the progress of the diet of the other's wife, with the response being, "Just fine: she's disappeared."

I had been put off by Pattie's poundage, but I felt a lot worse about it having been removed from my proximity entirely. That plus the astronomical expense of Pattie's life in Boston induced us to reconsider the long-term efficacy of the separation. We were reunited in late November 1995, after three months of making the heart grow fonder, and have lived together since.

My little life lessons were just getting started, however. Pattie went from fat to fatter in the summer of 1997, when she became ill from lupus. She was not yet 40 years old. At this point, she started putting on weight in earnest, as a function of the terrifying chronic illness. At this point, my still-present concerns about her appearance (for mostly selfish reasons, as you can probably guess) were overwhelmed by the immediacy of her situation and the realization that we had to start worrying about health and stop worrying about weight. (The terms are not synonymous, and I have often raised the question that if "health" is an issue, as it always is, why we are even discussing "weight." We'll have a collection of little insights on that topic later in the book.)

My testosterone kicked into high gear as the caregiver role was added to my list of responsibilities. I became very, very impatient with the mechanical remarks by others, especially those whose so-called professions indicated they should have known better, that Pattie needed to lose weight or she would drop dead. On many such occasions, the pundit in question did not even bother to ascertain whether there was some overriding reason for Pattie's physical shape before beginning to blather. My efforts to deal with such hostility (and I have long since ceased to see how such speech could be regarded as motivated by anything but hostility) have been as zealous as those that any self-respecting young spouse would demonstrate.

We do make light of Pattie's situation on occasion, and have applied for post-baccalaureate credit in gallows humor based on our work in that field. However, it has also been a serious matter, as certain elements of society have decided that the weakest of rationalizations will do to justify opening fire (if only metaphorically so to date) on my intelligent, spirited, and courageous wife.

The subject of this book is exactly how weak those rationalizations are, and exactly how pernicious is the notion that authority supersedes the need for any kind of accuracy in these cases. My co-author calls this narrative her personal story, but trust me, my co-author never wrote a story in her life without doing the background research first.

You may be wondering why I am a co-author or, more accurately, collaborator on this book. I have played three roles in the telling of this story.

First, I have been an honored witness to the events that are outlined in this book. I have watched Pattie struggle with self-acceptance, stigmatization, chronic illness and all the baggage that being fat in a society that hates fat and being ill in a society that hates disability carries. As with all good storytelling experiences, witnesses add flavor and legitimacy to the telling.

Second, I bring to the background research some knowledge of organizational studies, business, marketing, mathematics, statistics, media studies and philosophy. My formal and my independent education contributed much to the "making sense" part of this storytelling.

Finally, language is perhaps the most important part of storytelling. Getting the words right takes time, and often requires negotiation between two people. I have played the role of collaborator as we have together sought to find the right words to do justice to this story and its analysis. Pattie and I have collaborated often through exchanges of language. We co-produced an Internet talk show called *Coffee Shop* and an FM radio show called *First Person, Plural,* in both of which our trademark was bantering about ideas without the usual radio requisite of perpetual dumbing-down. The process of collaboration on this book was much the same as our radio experiences.

The story you are about to read is a well-thought-out tale that we hope will inspire you to consider both process and content. In short, we hope you learn something that will lead to the kind of growth we have experienced individually and as a couple as we have lived this story.

Carl
March 2005

Acknowledgements

Writing a book is never an individual or even team endeavor. It is always hard to tell where the book ends and the world begins, or vice versa. A lifetime of influences and experiences have contributed to this book, with thousands of people to thank.

Life is like that.

The whole point of this book is that none of us live in a social vacuum. So in a way, all those people who have taunted us, stared at us, treated us with disdain and refused to acknowledge us as human beings have contributed to this story. We are not grateful to them, but rather are grateful to those who have made it possible for us to endure stigma and to do so with grace and dignity. It is that social support we wish to acknowledge at this time.

Many stigmatized groups have cohesive networks and cultural commonalities that provide social support to endure prejudice and ostracism. Fat people often do not have such social support. Writing this book was made possible by a group of people who are trying to build such networks and cultures for people who accept fatness as simply an adjective rather than an indictment.

Specifically, we'd like to thank several friends we have made online and in person. Dana Schuster made us feel so welcomed when we visited San Francisco, and through her efforts we met with Marilyn Wann and

Lisa Tealer for a great afternoon's discussion that helped shape many of our thoughts while writing this book. We were especially happy to meet Marilyn, as her book, *FAT!SO?* was instrumental on our road to fat acceptance. We are grateful for Dana's work with the San Francisco Think Tank and for all the members of the Think Tank's e-mail list for their discussion and dedication to fighting for fat acceptance.

We also were privileged to spend some time with Deb Burgard, including a great time at her swimming pool on a warm May evening. Deb's longtime dedication to the health and well-being of fat people, as well as her intelligent analysis of the social contexts to that health and well-being, are inspirational. We have called on her several times during the production of this book, and she has been there every time with information and support, taking time out from her busy schedule for an e-mail or a phone call. We are also grateful for Deb Burgard's work creating and maintaining the "Show Me the Data" e-group. Without this community of scholars dedicated to critiquing obesity science and promoting Health at Every Size, our research for this book would have been considerably harder. There are literally hundreds of people on this e-mail list who have contributed to our understanding and analysis of the stigma of obesity. We apologize for not being able to name all of them.

We are specifically indebted to Paul Ernsberger and Glenn Gaesser and their continued dedication to translating the epidemiological and scientific data into chunks that are easier to understand for those of us who haven't spent years in the laboratory. While we made an effort to avoid making this a "health" book, having access to their knowledge and writings helped us sort out fact and science from fiction and hype.

Jon Robison's wit and insights were also influential. We share Jon's enthusiasm for Fritjof Capra's work and his understanding that science does not live a social vacuum, either. Jon's anger and outrage at the ways in which this culture have hurt fat people, and indeed anyone with a body, has been a source of inspiration and comfort over the three years in which we have exchanged e-mails both on-list and off-list.

Pat Ballard, Miriam Berg, Natalie Boero, Deb Burgard, Claudia Clark, Veronica Cook-Euell, Shari Dworkin, Jay Gubrium, Karin Kratina, Kathleen LeBesco, Paul McAleer, Tish Parmeley, and Sandy

Szwarc took the time to read the book before it was published and to provide feedback and support. Both were valued more than we can express.

Several friends and family put up with the obsession that becomes writing a book and listened warmly as we worked through the effort. Some have even provided us a place to stay during our travels, and financial support of our projects. Our gratitude to Peg Ainsley, Sylvia Ansay, Kelly Bliss, Kell Brigan, Lori Clarke, Floella Dobbs, Shelda Eggers, Cinder Ernst, Elaine Gallagher, Peggy Griffin, Susan Koppelman, Stef Maruch, Dennis Mills, Robin Mingle, and LaVelle Thomas for listening and being there not only throughout the writing of this book, but through the living of this story.

A special "thank you" to Danielle Provencher, who proofread the booklet "Before and After" over 10 years ago, and for her continued friendship since then. Also to Etta Breit, teacher extraordinaire, who encouraged Pattie in her writing about her life and experiences as a fat woman in a wonderful course called "Women's Bodies, Women's Minds." Without Etta's dedication to going the extra distance as a university instructor, many of the ideas in this book would have taken a lot longer to discover and develop.

A special "thank you" to Stephen Thomas, brother par excellence, our partner in crime—er, business—and the photographer behind many of the pictures in this book, as well as the technician who fixed many of the difficulties of moving material back and forth across the web. More than our "evil" twin, he has been the number one fan and the gadget man.

Several authors deserve special mention because they are highly influential on this work: specifically, Donileen Loseke and Jim Holstein for their important perspectives on social problems; Hernan Vera and Joe Feagin for their understanding of prejudice and the costs of racism, classism and sexism; George Ritzer for his excellent understanding of consumption in our society; and Sandra Harding for her work on the cultural context of scientific knowledge.

Three influential writers who are no longer with us, but from whom we have gleaned invaluable insights: Audre Lorde, who taught us to speak out; Michel Foucault, who taught us that the past is always understood in the present; and Erving Goffman, who taught us the cost of stigma and the price of "passing" in our presentation of self.

Perhaps our greatest influence sociologically, however, has been Jay Gubrium, who led Pattie's dissertation committee at the University of Florida and is now chair of the Department of Sociology at the University of Missouri at Columbia. Jay taught us in his classes, his writings and his personal discussions to understand the life course, selves and society with an eye for the nuances and complexities that the social life offers. Jay has also taught us through his example that justice and truth are often found in the details rather than grand narratives. Pattie has chosen a non-traditional post-doctoral path, and Jay has been supportive of that path wherever it has led. We are grateful for his guidance over the years, for his unquestioning support, and for his hospitality when we traveled through mid-Missouri for a short stay the summer of 2004.

In addition to San Francisco's "Our Think Tank" and the "Show Me the Data" e-mail lists, we have interacted with a number of people through several online forums including "Big Fat Blog," "Fat Studies," FAT!SO?'s "Gab Café," "Fatshadow," and all the wonderful people who have shown support through visiting, commenting and e-mailing us at "Fattypatties" (Pattie's blog for three years of working through the war on fat). We are grateful for all the interaction these forums have provided, and wish we could list every single one of the people who have shown us support and taught us so much over the years.

Also influential are the online opportunities we've had through sociological forums, including Sociologists for Women in Society (SWS) and the Sociology of Consumption group. Also, the guests and listeners and visitors to our *Cultural Construction Company* website and our sociological radio show, *First Person, Plural.*

Not many books have a mascot, but we want to especially acknowledge our cat, Anawim, who is a KWD (kitty with disabilities—she has a disorder similar to cerebral palsy in humans). Anawim has bravely traveled the world with us as we worked towards universal access in travel and researched

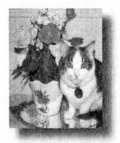

Anawim

this book. She doesn't like to travel, but she does tolerate it, and she certainly makes the trip more fun. We are honored to be allowed in her life.

A special "thanks" goes to Paul Campos. We had the privilege of interviewing him before his book *The Obesity Myth* was released, and while we were never able to air the interview on the radio, we were able to publish it on "Big Fat Blog." Then one May morning we took a detour through Boulder, Colorado and got to have breakfast with him. On the basis of this and an online exchange of thoughts and ideas, he generously offered to read the book and write our foreword. We are grateful for his support and for his continued work on behalf of fat people. We find him to be a kindred spirit who has little tolerance for injustice and stupidity and yet has great compassion for the victims of both. We are honored to have him as part of this effort.

Finally, we would like to acknowledge Peggy Elam, our editor and the owner of Pearlsong Press. Peggy has believed in this project from the beginning, and her dedication and insights have made this a better book than we could have ever done without her. But over the past year and a half Peggy has also become a friend. We are even more grateful for that privilege.

Our apologies to those we surely have forgotten.

Cheers,
Pattie & Carl
June 2005

All things appear and disappear
because of the concurrence of causes and conditions.
Nothing ever exists entirely alone;
everything is in relation to everything else.

A lesson from Buddha,
the original fat man with an attitude.

-- A Tale to Tell about Taking Up Space

I am about to tell a tale
I'm not supposed to speak.

"Before" Body Size Calculus:
The more space a body occupies,
the less knowledge a body has to offer.

> Only *afters* can tell this tale
> And I am a *before*.
> Because I take up space.

> > (Never mind that I have been an *after*
> > And a *before*
> > And another *after*
> > And another *before*
> > And a *during.*)

I will tell a tale,
I will speak.

"After" Body Size Calculus:
The space a body occupies
has nothing to do with the knowledge the body has to offer.

> *Befores* can tell this tale
> And I am a *before*.
> Because I take up space.

> > (Never mind that it is *after* my graduation
> > And *before* I see Antarctica
> > And *after* I learned to love my own skin
> > And *before* I take my first hot balloon ride,
> > And *during* my adventure called living.)

I take up space.
I move with grace.
I know my place.

I tell tales.

Pattie Thomas
2004

Body Size Calculus

Taking Up Space is a collection of essays, poems, narratives, photos and drawings that tell the story of my own intellectual, emotional and physical journey to fat acceptance.

The expression "fat acceptance" is a difficult phrase for many people. For some, it implies accepting a defect that has both physical and moral implications. For others, it is a question of aesthetics, not acceptance.

In popular discourse, "fat" is a noun that describes the very essence of the fat. A person *is* unconditionally fat, and a fat person *is* unconditionally ugly, lazy, unhealthy, and disgusting.

I have learned to regard fat as a description, a simple characteristic of the human body. Unfortunately, for me and for many people like me, the word "fat" comes with baggage. Fat acceptance is about examining that baggage and asking new questions about generally accepted ideas. Fat acceptance is about looking at the human body with different glasses. Fat acceptance is about removing a stigma that hurts not only the stigmatized, but a stigma that hurts all humans.

I have been told I was fat since the age of 11, when I gained 10 pounds over summer vacation, had to buy size "13-junior-petite" clothing, and subsequently attempted the first of many attempts to lose weight. I was never quite able to get to the ideal weights first expressed in life insurance charts and then in the pseudoscientific formula called the Body Mass Index (BMI). Even in my thinnest moments as an adult, I was considered fat.

Most of my life I have felt like I was at war with my own body. My body seemed out of control, and I spent huge amounts of effort, time and money to tame my appetites and contain my body into a thin version of itself. I have paid a huge physical and emotional price for those battles.

About 10 years ago, I began to suspect that the battle should not be fought within my self. Since that time, I have earned a Ph.D. in sociology. As a result, I have given a lot of thought to how social and cultural practices give contexts to our experiences as people.

I came to believe that I was engaged in a cultural struggle, not a medical one. Over the past 10 years, I slowly came to the realization that my body was okay and that, far from some internal conflict, the battles I had fought were in a war that was being waged *on* me and other people like me, and, to some extent, on us all.

In 1994, as part of an undergraduate class called "Women's Bodies/Women's Minds," I wrote a booklet called *Before and After: Living Fat in a Thin Society*, in which I addressed 10 myths about fatness. This booklet was the beginning of my journey to fat acceptance and being comfortable in my skin.

At first I was afraid to talk about my experiences as a fat woman. Then I read the following in an article on women's health:

> No one has been interested in the overweight woman's description of her own experience on the grounds that she must not know anything, otherwise she would be in better shape. Such a woman is presumed to be able to speak with authority only after she has lost weight. Until that time, describing her situation is considered to be a delaying tactic—her substitute for action.[1]

I realized that in a world where fat is something that is not desirable and getting thin is the ultimate achievement, the convention is that the only people with the authority to talk about their fatness are those who have lost their fatness. Asking a fat person about their lived experience is perceived as tantamount to legitimizing a drunk's excuses, thus ensuring that he or she keeps drinking.

Only the reformed drunk may tell his or her story with authority. Only "after" tales are legitimate, because the person telling the tale has been proven worthy through redemption and conformity.

I understood that I was *not* supposed to tell my story until I lost weight. I knew the source of my own fear.

When I read the above quote for the first time, I felt the sense of freedom and relief that comes from knowing what one needs to do next. I knew I needed to tell my story because I needed to demonstrate to myself that I could tell my story as a fat woman. I did not have to wait until I lost weight to speak.

The act of writing the booklet was a powerful experience. The reproduction of the booklet and its subsequent acceptance was also a powerful experience. What surprised me most was the number of women who were not fat, but understood the power of a fat woman talking about her body. I found that almost every woman I knew had a problem with her body—an unspeakable problem. In some way or another they felt unacceptable or ugly.

The power of a woman with a fat body talking about the unspeakable went beyond the issue of body size. It spoke to the depths of a consumption culture dependent upon human beings being perpetually dissatisfied with their physicality, with themselves.

A fat woman willing to talk about fat is a powerful thing.

The first section of this book is largely an updated rewrite of that booklet I wrote 10 years ago. I have updated what I wrote then to reflect what I have learned since then, but starting with these 10 myths was a good beginning to my journey and seems to be a good beginning to the telling of my journey.

I needed to challenge these myths in order to learn fat acceptance. I came to the conclusion that fat didn't have the power over my life that I had always thought it had held.

Before I came to this conclusion, I believed that I lacked will-power and was in need of fixing or curing. Essentially, I believed that my weight and body shape reflected a mental and moral imbalance. I thought that either I was trying to make up for some emotional problem or I was just lazy.

After I came to this conclusion, I saw my weight in light of my cultural environment. I am a product of the pressures to be thin, of the threats of violence in a society that keeps women in their place, and of the need to seek a powerful presence in a society that disenfranchised me for being a poor, working class woman.

It was only later that I also saw my weight as a product of my genetic makeup. Thus, this "after" turned out to be a "before" as well.

After writing *Before and After*, I still continued to try to lose weight. I told myself that I did so as a choice.

I stopped many of the really unhealthy practices I had used in the past. I didn't take drugs or supplements to lose weight. I tried more sensible approaches. I exercised regularly. I rode a bike or walked often. I counted calories and/or fat grams. I tried to eat more naturally, learning when I felt hunger and when I felt full. I examined and reexamined what emotional issues might have to do with my weight.

I did all these things, and I still couldn't lose weight for long without gaining it all back, plus some.

Then I got very sick. It took me almost six months to be diagnosed with what turned out to be systemic lupus erythematosus and fibromyalgia syndrome. Once I was diagnosed, a few more months passed before I was well enough to return to my daily activities. I was virtually bedridden for nine months. It also took some time to learn to live with a chronic, incurable condition. My ability to move around and do things was limited, and remains limited, to some extent. During this period, I got fatter.

As I got fatter and more disabled, I noticed a distinct change in attitudes towards me. I have always been the target of ridicule by strangers, even when I was small. Kids in school couldn't resist calling me "Fatty Patty" even when I was a skinny little kid. As I grew, the teasing became harassment. But during the first few years I was ill,

I noticed more and more people shunning me. It was no longer the occasional bully or routinely insensitive kid, it was colleagues and superiors showing a lack of respect for my work or utter shock when they discovered I could think and speak reasonably well.

Until the 1990s, I had always been a healthy fat person. Even doctors would say that the only thing that was wrong with me was my weight. My heart, my blood pressure, and my blood sugar were distinctly healthy. Moreover, I was quite successful on most of my weight loss efforts. I probably lost close to a thousand pounds, cumulatively, through various methods over the years. Frequently, these efforts led to some sort of physical breakdown like an injury, an infection, or an imbalance in electrolytes that ended the weight loss effort.

I was the quintessential weight-cycling dieter, and my efforts included harsh methods like starvation, drugs, laxatives and obsessive exercise. When the physical breakdown led to the necessary abandonment of the method, every loss was followed by the inevitable gain of even more weight. By the 1990s, I had done permanent damage to my health. No one knows why people get lupus, but I suspect that the abuse I put on myself in endless efforts to lose weight was part of the trigger mechanism that led to the onset of lupus.

However, health was never the real the motivation for me. My motivation for losing weight was almost always cosmetic in nature. I wanted to be thinner for a party, or a friend's wedding, or so I could fit into a smaller bathing suit. I thought of myself as ugly, and had little trust for men who found me attractive.

Of course, I had a "pretty face." Everyone said so. But only weight loss brought on fully enthusiastic compliments (or at least those were the only compliments I believed). The "fact" that fat was unhealthy was just extra motivation to help me achieve beauty.

I, of course, was not alone in connecting beauty with health. Go into any pharmacy or discount store in the United States or Canada and you will see a section called "Health and Beauty." Why?

When one sits down and thinks about it, what possible connection could health and beauty have? The answer, simply, is the human body. Within the confines of the health and beauty section are thousands of products claiming to change the body in some supposedly and particularly appealing way.

In our culture, fatness sits at the center of this intersection. The second section of this book examines that intersection.

Being fat is considered both unhealthy and ugly. Curing or making-over fatness is a multi-billion-dollar-a-year industry,[2] and it stands as one of the most workable arrangements under modern capitalism.

According to current economic rhetoric, the value of a product is derived from the extent of the desire for that product. As long as consumers want something, it is valuable, so the theory goes. Once the consumer is satisfied, the product loses value. Therefore, a product that is constantly desirable but never satisfies creates a sustainable demand.

The health and beauty industry loves fatness for exactly that reason. Cures and makeover techniques are rarely successful in making people thinner for a substantial length of time, and may even make people fatter. So people are encouraged to increase their desire for these products with each failed attempt to lose weight, and the seemingly perpetual capitalist machine continues.

Key to this dissatisfaction is a perpetually narrowing view of health and a perpetually narrowing view of beauty. If definitions of health and definitions of beauty were broadened to include fatness, the hold this industry has on people of all sizes would be loosened.

For a long time, I measured myself according to these narrower visions. I also measured others. I was sympathetic to people who were different from the ideal, but I didn't see them as beautiful. Then one day, I was riding the bus on the way to class and I asked myself what beauty was.

As a photographer, I had learned a lot about light and shadow. I knew that the "perfect" models filling magazines looked perfect because a light shone on them directly from the front.

Go through any fashion magazine and look at the eyes of the models in the ads. Around the pupil of their eyes you will usually see a ring of light reflected. This is from the light that circles the lens on the camera taking the picture. A bright light hitting an object directly casts no shadow visible to the camera and creates the illusion of flatness. So even before the inevitable airbrushing, any blemishes, any wrinkles, and/or any imperfections disappear under the gaze of the hard, bright light.

As a photographer, I knew the ideal was an illusion, a trick of shadow and light. But on that bus, that particular morning, I decided to look at each person on the bus and to ask myself where her or his beauty lay. To my surprise, I found something beautiful about each person on the bus. By beauty, I mean something appealing about the way they looked physically. I do not mean that I speculated on some inner quality.

Can people just change their minds about their tastes? Advertisers seem to believe that they can shape our thinking and tastes. My exercise in people-watching changed the way I looked at people. These things suggest that, indeed, it is possible to examine tastes and perceptions, questioning them and reshaping them to new evaluations.

In the late 1960s, during the Civil Rights Movement, the slogan "Black is Beautiful" became a popular affirmation of African-American bodies, styles and traditions. The Afro, or "going natural," was a visible affirmation of Black beauty. This was not a simple exercise in self-esteem. It was a political statement, and it led to changes in the manufacturing and promotion of a number of products from toys to hair care to beer.

There can be no fat acceptance until there is an appreciation of the beauty of fat and fat people.

I personally found that it was not until I appreciated the beauty of others that I became comfortable with my own beauty. I still have "ugly days" on which I feel like I must be awful to behold. But learning to see the beauty in others and questioning the standards offered me was an important part of my journey to fat acceptance.

My journey has not ended with acceptance of my own beauty. I stopped dieting around the time that my ideas about beauty changed. I began to understand myself as born fat. I saw my attempts to lose weight as attempts to "pass" for thin. I started accepting myself as a fat person and started working on being the healthiest person I could be, making fat irrelevant to that quest.

My personal transformations are not enough. A number of economic interests exist to "fix" people like me, and these interests don't just evaporate because I feel better about myself.

Fat acceptance is about a larger context. As long as fat is regarded as a disease, fat acceptance will be compromised. The medicalization of fat is the key to keeping fat hatred in place and leaving it unchallenged.

The rhetoric of health care workers and government officials has turned nasty in the past few years. Like the "war on drugs," the new agenda is a "war on obesity," and my new awareness of how manipulating the environment can be has made me acutely aware of how hostile the culture has become towards fat people.

Simply identifying cultural, political and economic perceptions that create popular beliefs about fat people is not enough to create change. These perceptions are marbled through the culture, and there are some powerful incentives for these perceptions to be supported and sustained.

In 1963, sociologist Erving Goffman, in his seminal work *Stigma*, outlined the social interaction between people who are perceived as "normal" and people who are perceived as "spoiled." The current language of the "war on obesity" that can be found in western cultures around the world is reminiscent of Goffman's descriptions.

Fat people are not regarded simply as a group of people with a medical condition. Their *identity* is inextricably tied to being fat. Being fat in a world that considers fatness abnormal means being perceived as spoiled. Thus, the "war on obesity" is actually a war not on a disease, but on the people who are considered to have that disease. The war on obesity is a war on fat people.

For fat people, especially those of us who have a positive and accepting view of ourselves and other fat people, such a war is disturbing. We find ourselves reluctant warriors in a war that we did not start and we do not want to fight.

If the stigma of fatness is to be removed, first the stigma must be taken from the minds and hearts of those who believe that fat is ugly, fat is unhealthy, fat is bad. However, to be truly successful in removing the stigma of fatness, the methods of "fixing" fatness must lose their profitability.

Joe McVoy, an eating disorders specialist and co-founder of the now-defunct Association for the Health Enrichment of Large People (AHELP), called the multi-billion dollar weight-loss industry the "diet-pharmaceutical industrial complex."[3] These industries include extremely lucrative businesses that command high sales, extremely well-funded research and development laboratories that receive large government and pharmaceutical research grants, and extremely popular counseling and advice services that maintain high profiles in mass media markets.

As long as such economic interests remain profitable, fat stigma will be perpetuated. As long as those who control popular discourse define and require others to define fatness as a disease called "obesity," these interests will be sustained. Fighting this war begins with questioning the validity of the medical condition called "obesity."

There once was a time when scientists believed that the size of one's forehead could predict criminal behavior and that the bumps on one's head could reveal personality characteristics. Perfectly acceptable medical opinions by the "standards" of their respective contemporary medical establishments asserted that women could not be educated because the blood-letting that occurred during menstruation drained the brain of blood, making women intellectually inferior to men. Race was believed to have a biological basis, with light skin being correlated to evolutionary superiority. All of these absurd ideas were studied and substantiated "scientifically" until they fell out of favor.

Someday, the term "obesity" will be an anachronism, and "fatness" will be just another adjective, as benign as "tallness" or "darkness." In such a fat-neutral world the health and beauty of all people will be acceptable, not under attack, and appreciated.

The third section of this book comes from my reflection on fighting this war on "obesity." In a way, I have come full circle.

I began my journey towards fat acceptance by giving up a war that I was fighting with my own body, and coming to an understanding that a cultural context exists to my feelings about my body and the bodies of others. Of late, the cultural war has heated up, and the current climate is creating a great deal of stress for fat people like me. I have come to regard some physical environments as hostile, especially those that provide no appropriate seating for larger people or set up barriers to our entrance.

In December of 2002, I was hospitalized for bacterial pneumonia. Fighting off infections is difficult for people with lupus because both the disease and the treatments affect the immune system. As a fat person, I hate medical encounters. No matter what symptoms or health problems I face, my body size is going to be an issue, and it makes trusting medical advice—well, complicated.

During my hospitalization, while I was lying in a bed, hooked to oxygen and having a hard time breathing, much less talking, a doctor took the opportunity to lecture me on how I needed to lose weight. I responded weakly and between gasping breaths that I no longer made efforts to lose weight. I whispered that I was willing to exercise and even change my diet, but I was not willing to make weight loss a goal.

I was ambushed, and because I was too sick to respond, I made little progress in heading off the lecture that ensued. However, one interesting comment came from the physician's lecture, and it served to change the way I thought about my body and about being a warrior in the war on fat people. In response to my albeit weak assertion that I no longer tried to lose weight, the doctor said, "Yes, it is true that some people can carry their weight well, but this pneumonia shows that you are not one of those people."

He may have meant his statement to motivate me to lose weight, which probably justified, in his mind, his ambushing me in the first place. But as I lay in the hospital bed contemplating his words, it occurred to me that a second option was open. *What if I trained my body to carry my weight well?*

Losing weight is not the answer, because it is rarely a successful strategy in the long run. My personal history showed me that I would only end up getting fatter, and even worse, sicker.

But the doctor might be right, after a fashion. Maybe there *were* people who carried their weight well. What would I need to do to become one of those people?

Before getting sick in 1997, I had done weight training, lifting free weights and using some pulley machines. I learned from my trainer that kinesiologists consider five components for fitness: strength, flexibility, stamina, balance, and body composition. Weight training contributes directly to the first four components and supposedly helps indirectly with the fifth, because, theoretically, stronger and more flexible muscles increase metabolism and supposedly burn fat. I am not convinced of the validity of the fat-burning theory, but I do think that body composition could figure into an optimal formula for fitness.

In a fat-neutral world where being fat was not considered to be unconditionally bad, it might make sense for people of different sizes to exercise their bodies differently. Wouldn't it be wonderful, I mused, to be taught how to *carry my weight* rather than fight it? What would I need to do so?

The answer, for me, has been to increase my strength, flexibility, stamina and balance through exercise.

Since getting back into the gym and becoming stronger, I have started noticing fat athletes. Football, baseball, hockey, and even basketball have their share of large people. While most of these athletes are men, there are women wrestlers and softball players who are fat and competitive.

Few of these athletes are very fat, and many who are considered big are really not that much bigger than the average man or woman. However, fat athletes who are very fat and who use their fat in their sport do exist: male and female sumo wrestlers.

The Sumo is also interesting because the sport is derivative of the legendary Samurai. The Sumo is not only a fat athlete; he or she is a fat *warrior*. The ritual that takes place before a sumo wrestling match represents the warrior code passed down to ensure that the mind and body of the warrior are prepared for attack.

The Sumo is an incredible symbol for fat people upon whom war is being waged. In the war on fat people, I want to be a Sumo Warrior, prepared to defend my people, my mind, my body and my soul.

The Sumo, like their contemporary counterparts, the Marines, were the first line of defense in war. It was their job to make a path through enemy ranks that would allow the army behind them to make progress and gain territory.

Fat people are the first line of defense in a political economy designed to make all people feel dissatisfied with their bodies and then exploit that dissatisfaction for profit. Fat people are the first line of defense in a culture built upon a glorification of impossibly narrow standards of beauty and health.

Acceptance of fat people will open up possibilities of recognition and acceptance of the beauty and the healthiness of *all* bodies. As we open up spaces for ourselves, fat people can open up spaces and make room for everyone. I believe fat acceptance can lead to a market based upon accepting the wonderful diversity of human bodies instead of making profits based upon dissatisfaction and fear.

The fat warrior is fighting for a more just political economy in which everyone would benefit.

Taking Up Space is written in two voices: my professional knowledge and my personal experiences.

As a sociologist, I offer reasonable arguments about social and cultural forces that reinforce hurtful ideas about fatness and limit the life chances of fat people. I have studied stigma and the consequences of stigma both through reading sociological literature and doing original research. I am a medical sociologist and have studied medical systems and the social roles played within those systems through reading medical literature and doing original research. I cannot help but bring that knowledge to bear on my understanding of fatness. I do not intend to write a sociological treatise on the subject of fat acceptance, but I do intend to stand on the authority from my training and expertise.

Make no mistake, however; I take the war on fat people personally. I do not leave my home without having to anticipate seating arrangements, spatial limitations, potential harassment, and well-intentioned insults. I am never sure if any medical advice I seek, a particular professional treatment of my work, or the normal ebb and flow of my personal relationships are being tainted by negative attitudes about my body. I live with the stress of this stigma every day. It is pervasive and constant.

As a person living with chronic illness, I find this stigma to be doubly painful. Not only do I believe that my disability was, in part, created because of my 20-year struggle to fight fat, but it remains complicated by the stigma I experience as both a fat person and a disabled person. I believe that my personal experience with daily facing stigma gives me a perspective on social relationships that can be useful to others.

This is a personal journey, and I stand on the authority of my personal and professional experience. All too often fat and disabled people are discussed by experts who have not taken the time to consider the consequences of their words.

In addition to essays and reasoned arguments, I have included poetry, stories, photos and drawings. I have included these things because other fat people might see themselves in my experience, and they may be encouraged. I have included these things because the central function of creating a social stigma is to reinforce the idea that people of certain groups are not human beings.

I am an intelligent, deeply feeling, creative and artistic human being. Most people see me as fat before they see me as any of those things. Erving Goffman summed up this social interaction best in his description of "normals" versus "spoiled" people:

> The attitudes we normals have toward a person with a stigma, and the actions we take in regard to him, are well known, since these responses are what benevolent social action is designed to soften and ameliorate. *By definition, of course, we believe the person with a stigma is not quite human.* On this assumption we exercise varieties of discrimination, through which we effectively, if often unthinkingly, reduce his life chances.

Ending this war on the "obese" requires changes of heart, changes of economy, changes of politics, and changes of culture. My hope is that by recognizing the beauty and strength of fat people, we can come to see ourselves and be seen by others as the wonderful people we are and we can become.

Before and After

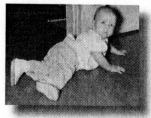

Seven months old

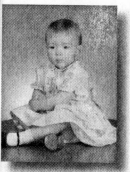

Two years old

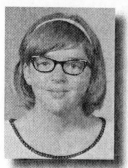

Age 11, going on 16.
Went on first diet
because I looked
"so fat."

— Before and After

BEFORE:

When I was a child
    (they told me i was ONLY a girl)
I talked like a child
    (too much, they said, "SHUT UP")
I thought like a child
    (why? why? why? why? why? why? why? why? WHY?)
I reasoned like a child
    (it must be me, i'm NOT enough)

When I became a (wo)man
    (a GOOD girl)
I put childish things behind me
    (and knew my PLACE)

Now we see through a glass darkly
    (for i am lost even to my own reflection)
But then we shall see face to face
    (how will i reclaim my image?)

AFTER:

> and now these three
> > (childlike)
> things remain:

> faith
> > (in who i am)
> hope
> > (in who i can become)
> love
> > (the most childlike thing of all)

> but the greatest of these is
> love
> > (i learned to love me again)

Pattie Thomas
1994
(An adaptation of Paul's letter to the Christians at Corinth
in the first century, CE)

*I have come to believe
over and over again
that what is most important to me
must be spoken,
made verbal and shared,
even at the risk
of having it bruised
or misunderstood.*

Audre Lorde

The Diet Ends (Begins) —

hot salsa burns my stomach, betraying
yet another binge of mexican magic
leaving me hung over
without a
drop of liquor and
(god, my head hurts)
i am afraid
that i have done
damage again.

why can't i get it through
my head that i
am going to die from this food
from this eating

please, god, don't let me die . . .
fat

i wonder if that is gas or a heart attack?

tomorrow
i will do better
i will exercise
i will starve myself to make up for yesterday (today)
i will be thin

let us
see if
i eat only
lettuce
for the next 3
months i
will lose
40 pounds of ugly fat
(and some muscle tissue, possibly organ tissue
and other minor things)
and i will feel better (thinner)

please pass me the croissant and hot cocoa
i'm too tense to start today

Pattie Thomas
1994

> *Myth #1: Fat is unhealthy.*
>
> *There is a good deal of evidence indicating that many of the more prevalent weight-related health problems, such as high blood pressure, elevated cholesterol and triglyceride levels, insulin resistance, and glucose intolerance, can be improved independently of weight loss.*
>
> Glenn Gaesser, Ph.D.
> exercise physiologist & author of *Big Fat Lies*

Many years ago, my internist told me about a family of extremely "overweight" people. The mother, father, and daughter each weighed over 400 pounds. Mom and Dad were in their 70s, and their daughter was in her 50s. The doctor said that, in all honesty, he found it difficult to tell them they should lose weight, because they had genetically high HDL (the good cholesterol) and probably could live to be over 100.

"Weight isn't really the problem," he confided in me. "It is high blood counts of LDL cholesterol, high blood pressure, and high blood sugar (indicating diabetes) that are the culprits. Weight control is only good if you lower those indices in the process."

Then, even though I had no problems, nor had I ever *had* any problems, with any of these indices, he gave me a prescription for diet pills, to which I subsequently became addicted.

Medical anthropologist Cheryl Ritenbaugh studied obesity and the biomedical establishment's treatment of obesity in relationship to western societal values. She found that in the 20th century, as thinness became a more desirable beauty standard, the biomedical practitioners' research and treatment of obesity rose in prominence. Ritenbaugh found that "the changing biomedical standards have paralleled changing cultural values, rather than an accumulation of biomedical knowledge."

Diabetes, high blood pressure, heart disease and a fat body type seem to be connected in some way, but scientists far from understand the connection. The relationship between fat and disease remains more controversial than corporate media infoganda headlines would lead one to believe. Being large can put an extra burden on movement, but many times physical restrictions have more to do with one-size-fits-all engineering than with a large person's body and health. What seems to be more important is eating healthy food and exercising regularly.

While the jury is still out on the role of fatness in good health, many physicians have the same prejudices as others in society, neglecting to treat their fat patients' symptoms and opting instead to insist that weight loss is the answer to all their health problems. Many large people have trouble getting health care because insurance companies and employers discriminate on the basis of size.

The stress of living in a society that harasses and threatens fat people can *create* ill health. A person's health is hurt by fat most often from the prejudice of others.

Myth #2: Fat is mental illness.

Many obesity researchers believe that psychological problems cause many people to overeat and get fat. But [eating disorder researcher David] Garner turns their world view upside down: It's dieting, he says—along with the social stigma against fat people—that causes the psychological problems that many fat people, chronic dieters, and people with eating disorders experience. The fat people who don't diet, and who have learned to challenge the culture that tells them they're worthless because of their weight, simply don't have those psychological problems.

Laura Fraser
journalist & author of *Losing It*

According to the National Association of An-
orexia Nervosa and Associated Disorders, nearly eight million people suffer from at least one of the three main eating disorders (anorexia nervosa, bulimia, and binge eating disorder), and 90 percent of those suffering are women.

Most sufferers report onset by the age of 20, and most sufferers will spend at least five years of their lives in the throes of their disorders. All minorities groups and socio-economic levels are affected. An estimated 6 percent will die because of complications from these disorders, and only about 50 percent report that they are cured.[1]

Treatment of eating disorders lies primarily in the hands of mental health professionals. Along with these disorders, fat people are often treated for depression and nervous disorders solely on the basis of their being fat. The assumption that fat must be a symptom of mental illness in whomever it occurs has a long history, with a variety of therapies and treatments.

The truth about fat acceptance, however, may be very much the opposite of mental illness. The decision not to make weight loss a goal and to live as a fat person in a thin-obsessed society is a decision to come to terms with one's identity in that society. No doubt, psychological counseling for compulsive behaviors has been beneficial to some fat individuals. But it must be understood that to benefit from counseling does not prove that mental illness is present or that being fat has created and/or results from a mental disorder.

— Orderly Responses

OBSESSIVE/COMPULSIVE DISORDER
What's so unusual
about the worry I feel
about my body
in a world that is dangerous?
What's so unusual
about the compulsion
to protect myself?

POST TRAUMATIC STRESS DISORDER
I was only trying to cope
with the shame of his hands
upon my little body and the
fear that he
may come
again

BORDERLINE PERSONALITY DISORDER
Excuse me, but in this mundane
extremely stressful world of
hard demands on a
malleable soul
I many times
run away to
cry and
grieve

COMPULSIVE OVEREATING
Somehow, I think a better term might be
REPULSIVE OVEREATING
because this attraction
to the comfort of food
is directly proportional
to the repulsion
I feel
at (in) the world

CLINICAL DEPRESSION
How dare I be sad
in such a wonderful world
that invites me to
be myself on such
a regular
basis?

Pattie Thomas
1994

> ## Myth #3: Fat is unwanted.
>
> *Until the 1980s, excess weight was the target of most ads for diet products; today, one is much more likely to find the enemy constructed as bulge, fat, or flab. . . . To achieve such results (often envisioned as the absolute eradication of body, as in 'no tummy') a violent assault on the enemy is usually required; bulges must be 'attacked' and 'destroyed,' fat 'burned,' and stomachs (or more disgustedly, 'guts') must be 'busted' and 'eliminated.'*
>
> Susan Bordo
> cultural critic & author of *Unbearable Weight*

As I write this book, the private, nonprofit Ad Council—the primary creator of public service advertising campaigns in America—has begun a new campaign, sponsored by the U.S. Department of Health and Human Services, called "Small Steps." It includes three television public service announcements featuring severed body parts being left in public places.

A "belly" is found on a beach, "love handles" are found in a stairwell, and a "double chin" is found in the produce department at a grocery. The plot to the ads is that someone happens upon these severed body parts. Instead of being immediately repulsed, they explain the body part as having been "lost" there because the person to whom the part once belonged was walking, taking the stairs, or snacking on fruits and vegetables, respectively. The intent is to suggest that exercise and eating healthily will help people "shed" their fat.

"Shedding fat" plays on a long-standing rhetoric about diet, exercise and weight loss. The "Small Steps" campaign isn't the first time someone in the media has used fetishized images of human fat to represent the supposedly desirable goal of losing fat. Anyone born in or before 1980 and had access to American television can remember Oprah Winfrey and her little wagon of 67 pounds of fat that she brought out on stage to represent the weight she lost on the Optifast diet (or, more

M.C. Diet —

Atkins and Stillman
Milkshakes in a can
Grapefruit on the table
Sweets are contraband

High protein drinks
Nothing refined
Take three a day
And don't trust your mind

Eggs and pineapple
Burning ugly fat
Drink vinegar for breakfast
Then hit the floor mat

Ten food exchanges
Like money in your fist
Spent before the day's over
What did I pay for this?

Little pills made
To suppress my appetite
Make me energetic
Keep me up all night.

Shots of placenta
(Meant to help me diet)
Or Vitamin B-12
Just to keep me quiet

Pritikin soups are
Ummm, ummm, good
Herbal remedies
Taste like wood

Too many options
Willpower waning
Think I'll have a pizza
Screw maintaining

Pattie Thomas
1994

aptly nicknamed, "Optifamine"). They should also remember than she gained the weight back very rapidly, and that the diet has been controversial because of the damage it can do to the health of the dieter.

Marilyn Wann's playful lost-pound vacation photos in her book *FAT!SO?* is a wonderful commentary on shedding unwanted fat. Wann asks, "Where does a lost pound of fat go?" She then tells the tale, including pictures, of her lost pound of fat taking a global vacation during which it meets other pounds of fat. After a great trip, the lost pound and its friends come back home to be on your body where they belong. I've had a lot of lost pounds come back home with friends over the years.

Fat being unwanted is a concept that assumes fat is something other than one's *true* body. Fat cells, like all other naturally occurring cells in our bodies, are a necessary part of what keeps us alive and healthy. Losing weight and losing fat are not synonymous. Dieting and exercise might result in a smaller body (often they do not), but they never result in the loss of fat cells without the loss of other cells as well.

I want my fat in part because I want my body to be whole and to function the best it can.

I was not a regular watcher of the show *Saturday Night Live* by the 1990s, so Julia Sweeney's androgynous character "Pat" escaped my notice for some time, in spite of our common name. *It's Pat* was made into a feature film, and like all things pop cultural, the shtick found its way into my consciousness at some point. Specifically, I saw a scene from the film in which Pat falls in love. Finally, Pat's friends could know if Pat was a man or a woman, a question of considerable interest and debate. Pat's beau, Chris, however, turns out to be just as androgynous as Pat, and the mystery lives on.

What intrigued me most about Pat is that Julia Sweeney wears a fat suit in order to pull off the ruse of androgyny. Fat is frequently depicted as both unfeminine and non-masculine. Women who are fat violate a significant taboo against taking up space. Women of all sizes are taught to sit with legs or ankles crossed, elbows and arms tucked in nicely, taking up as small a space as possible. Men, on the other hand,

— on being a girl...

there are days
when i am five years old
(a hypocrite who acts grown up)

just a little girl
who wants to be held
and loved

there are days
when i am a powerful old woman
(a wise sage who acts childish)

just a big woman
who wants to be heard
and heeded

there are days
when i am a sexy vixen
(a buxom goddess who acts playful)

just a sensuous being
who wants to be touched
and satisfied

there are days
when i am a brilliant scholar
(an intuitive mind who acts thoughtfully)

just another smart person
who wants to be respected
and published

Pattie Thomas
1994

are allowed to expand their bodies and fill up the space around them. But fat men still do not meet gender expectations. Men who are fat violate the masculine taboo of softness. Men are supposed to be hard-bodied and strong. Fat symbolizes weakness.

Historian Peter N. Stearns notes that, in recent years, the push towards a hard and slender body found in advice for both genders can be seen as an attempt to desexualize and standardize bodies. Stearns writes, "In a broad sense, the widespread acceptance of this [anti-fat] culture is part of a longer-term standardization of the human body as well as the acceptance of constraint over spontaneous bodily impulses."[2]

Judging the femininity and masculinity of any person on the basis of their appearance limits the life chances of all people. The myth that fat is androgynous is the myth that people are either one gender or another, and that violation of that dichotomy is an aberration. Gender is better modeled as a continuum, with each person having a mixture of both. Even fat people.

Myth #5: Fat is asexual.

Consider for a moment the most ancient human images known: the intriguing Venus figures that date back twenty-five thousand years. . . . These relics depict a full-bodied female, her large, pendulous breasts spilling over a swollen abdomen, her mammoth thighs support a rotund rump. . . . Imagine a hominid hunter, far from home and lonely, fingering the curvaceous belly and breasts of a Venus figure for comfort and erotic pleasure.

Rita Freedman
feminist & author of *Beauty Bound*

I have been thin, and I have been fat, and I have had sexual relationships in both states of body.

Some men lost interest as I lost weight. Some men preferred me full-figured, with my breasts larger and my thighs and genitals more encompassing to enhance pleasure. More to the point, I have found sex pleasurable and fulfilling no matter what my body size. There have been advantages to being heavier as well as to being thinner.

The fact that no one really talks about fat people today in sensuous terms is indicative of societal norms that connect sexuality with thinness. This may not only be a myth, it might be in direct opposition to the truth. According to author Naomi Wolf in her book *The Beauty Myth,* "researchers at Michael Reese Hospital in Chicago found that plumper women desired sex more often than thinner women. On scales of erotic excitability and readiness, they outscored thin women by a factor of almost two to one."

The belief that thin is sexual is a pressure that is placed on both men and women of all sizes and sexual orientations. This belief influences not only the size we desire our bodies to be, but the size we desire our partners to be. The truth is that while our culture esteems one body type over another in different historical periods (the voluptuous woman of the late '50s, the Twiggy flat chest of the '60s, the thin running man of the '70s, the pumped-up iron man of the '90s), people come in varieties at all times, and so do our tastes in sexual partners.

What is liberating for people of all sizes is the enjoyment of our own bodies. Poet Audre Lorde calls this deeply felt experience the power of the "erotic." She asserts that one of the tools of oppression is to teach us not to trust our bodies and our feelings. Erotic feelings are based on a combination of both our bodies and our emotions.

The myth of fat as asexual is the myth that people must have idealized bodies to experience pleasure. Nothing could be further from the truth.

--- *The Split* —

Like with a knife
cut in twos
Who am I?
What are the rules?

How do I stop
the voices within?
"Failure" (fat)
"Whore" (thin)

Tell the truth
of who I am
Afraid I can't
Afraid I can.

Pattie Thomas
1990

Myth #6: Fat is incompetent.

The linkage of health as well as appearance with slenderness, along with the larger impulse to use a slim body as a talisman of a good, well-disciplined character, supported another new theme in the campaign against fat—the association of weight control with work.

Peter N. Stearns
historian & author of *Fat History*

In 1993, in the United States, an appellate court

rendered a decision that essentially made being fat a "handicap." For too long, fat people—especially, though not exclusively, women—have been unable to get the job opportunities that thin people have. Among other reasons for this is the perception that fat people are incompetent, not able to perform well.

In our society, the myth of fat as incompetent is perpetuated by our ideal of "success." We are motivated by sayings such as "No pain, no gain," and "You can never be too rich or too thin." Thinness is a mark of success. Fatness is a mark of failure.

Communicologist Carole Spitzack speaks of a society that condemns women who exceed their prescribed boundaries. When we exceed those boundaries, we are called to a kind of confessional, a listing of our sins. Being fat, having a body that doesn't fit the prescription, is in essence a confession of sinfulness. Spitzack asserts that the very nature of dieting is confessional and even spiritual, with the hope of an "afterlife," a thin life:

> It is the vision of afterlife that sustains dieting vigilance. To succeed, she opposes the lives of fat women and thin women and resolves to make the transition from fat to thin. Images of afterlife characterized by overall spiritual and social health

demand a repeated condemnation of a woman's *present* body and present life."[3]

Calling obesity a handicap is a mixed blessing. It assumes that fat is a disease or condition that needs to be treated or changed rather than an adjective that describes the noun "person." Fat people do suffer from discrimination and prejudice, but they generally have more in common with visible minorities and homosexuals than they do with physically handicapped or disabled groups.

On one hand, fat people are visible, and their bodies are regarded as inferior simply because of the way they look. Like other visible minorities, much of the discrimination they face has more to do with how they look than who they are. On the other hand, fat people are believed to have control over their fatness and are therefore expected to conform to the norms and mores of what a "good" body should be. Like homosexuals, many fat people assert that they are expected to control or change something that is biological and genetic in nature, and an attempt to conform relies upon a denial of something fundamental about their identity.

Of course, it is true that accommodations are often needed in order for a fat person to be able to participate in daily activities. Spatial designs often assume a certain size body, and many fat people cannot fit in many one-size-fits-all spaces. Of course, similar accommodations are needed for left-handed people, shorter people, taller people, and some older people.

Perhaps, rather than deciding what rights a certain group has, the answer lies in respecting the dignity of all people and challenging the engineers and architects of the world to create designs with universal access.

— *Super Adorable People* *

When I sat
across the desk
from well-dressed
super adorable people (SAPs)
and asked for my livelihood,
I wondered if
all they saw was my
"out-of" shape?

When I took care
of the little children
of well-dressed
super adorable people (SAPs, jr.)
for my livelihood
I wondered if
all they saw were my
maternal looks?

Pattie Thomas
1994

* *A thank you to short-story writer Rosario Ferré for the term*
"super adorable people." "SAPs" are the best of the beautiful people.

Myth #7: Fat is jolly.

During my three years at NYU, I had developed elaborate defense mechanisms and an ordered system of self-reliance. Much of this, of course, was a façade. I was honing my lying skills as I perfected my acting skills. I was putting forth the image of the jolly fat girl to cover up a morass of self-hatred, despair, and deceit. I was defending the inner sanctum like a lion defends her cubs. Only I was a cub. I was told and I believed that it was my fault for being fat and that if I wanted to change it, I could.

Camryn Manheim
award-winning actress & author of *Wake Up! I'm Fat!*

Keeping a sense of humor is important in the

health and well-being of every person. Laughing at ourselves is a useful way to put things in perspective. I make "broad" jokes because I love the double entendre it conjures up and the fact that the word is even funnier coming from a "known" feminist and broadly fat woman.

Being able to laugh at ourselves, however, does not discount or resolve the pain that often comes with being fat in a society of people who value thinness. Our experience of being fat can define our lives and create tremendous pain. Psychologist Laura Brown writes about the self-hatred many women experience:

> Second only to the constant fear of physical and sexual assault . . . this self-hatred attached to body size and eating habits is a most pernicious source of energy drain for women. It serves as a patriarchal psychic tapeworm, eating away at energy and self-love and reducing women's abilities to act powerfully. Fat oppression is one form of discrimination that is still acceptable to practice, even in the feminist community.[4]

The myth of fat people being jolly is born in the practice of blaming victims for victimization. As fat people, we endure discriminatory practices.[5] Being the clown in social situations does not make up for these practices, or for the pain that these practices exact upon our lives and our life chances. In light of this, the expectation that we accept our lot with the grace of laughing at ourselves is anything but funny.

— Silhouettes

I walk in silent silhouettes
Through ghostly corridors.
I talk.
My mouth moves. My ears hear tones.
I carry on complete conversations.
I comprehend nothing.
I am detached, not really present.
I am not here.

I am only an observer.
I am possessed.
I feel nothing.
I don't even feel at peace,
Just nothingness,
Empty corridors of nothingness.
Emptiness.
Black darkness.

And life seems to have no purpose
Other than to go through the motions
and sleep.

Those of us who speak out about these discriminatory practices are often taken to task for "being too serious." We are labeled humorless and selfish when we refuse to endure jokes and teasing, but condescending humor further supports these discriminatory practices.

Fat people are capable of great humor, but the stigma fat people face every day is no laughing matter.

God, I wish I could sleep
Without the nightmares,
Without the dreams of hope.
I want my sleep to be as empty as my days.
Is there any reason, any rhythm for all this?

Depression you've come to visit again
And like mother, when you are here,
You take over.
Little pills to make me better.
I hate this life.
I hate being sick.
Being depressed makes me angry . . . and sad.

Just hang on; just stay together long enough.

Why the desperation?
Why the dis-ease?
Why the pain?
Why me?

Pattie Thomas
1989

Myth #8: Fat is bitchy.

Sometimes a private cry is what is needed. Give yourself the chance to feel those feelings, and then let them go. . . . Enjoy a good one-liner retort. It's fine to be a little 'naughty.'

Bonnie Bernell
psychologist & author of *Bountiful Women*

Often women are taught to be nice girls and never to express anger. While being allowed much more emotional expression than men, we are often punished for expressions of anger and sexuality. These are male domains, or, rather, *slender* male domains. Fat men are often regarded as slobs or goons because of their size. One only need note the rhetoric Michael Moore faced after his speech at the 2002 Oscars to see how fatness can be used as a signifier of unacceptable anger.

But women hold a special title for expressing their anger. Powerful women are called "bitches," often as a means to quiet them. It is no coincidence that when men are chastised for their anger they are called "sons of bitches" or "bastards," thereby implicating their mothers.

Power comes with anger, and therein lays the threat. Fat people often are said to be suppressing their anger by stuffing it with food. In fact, the opposite might be true. Accepting and celebrating our fat bodies may be an expression of both anger and power.

Fat people in touch with this power are formidable indeed, especially if they have found enough self-love to withstand the criticism that will surely fall their way. Poet Audre Lorde wrote about the uses of anger as a key mechanism to ensure survival in a world that intends on the destruction of certain people. With anger often comes clarity.

There is much about which fat people should be angry. We suffer discrimination. We suffer ridicule. We suffer loneliness and ostracism. Taking these things without emotional reaction is to learn powerless-ness. Anger can be used to reclaim ourselves and our right to be human. Anger can be a source of tremendous resistance to oppression.

The myth of bitchiness comes from the threat of power. Anger about fatness, by both women and men of all sizes, is an important component in the process to changing stigma, including the stigma that continues to oppress fat people.

———————————————————— *Ticked Off* —

Anger boils within me
Steaming, simmering,
Too hot to touch, I'm sure
Pressure is building up
Like my mother's steam cooker
It ticks off
chattering
e r r a t i c a l l y   r h y t h m a t i c

I am afraid.
Afraid of what?

If I get angry
I won't be loved?
Do I destroy with my
feelings?

Anxiety
Worry

I don't know what to do
DO
There must be something I can
DO

I find myself these days not only feeling,
but insisting on my RIGHT TO FEEL.

Like brown rice in a slow cooker,
I fill my space in fluffy swells
From hard grains I puff up to soft chewiness

Somehow I stopped regarding pain
as something to fight, to avoid.

Pressure built up like the steam cooker
Ticking off, chattering erratically.

I am mad.
No longer crazy, but angry.

Pattie Thomas
1989

Myth #9: Fat is lazy.

Common societal views portray obesity as a sign of contemptible self-indulgence and decadence that would be remedied by a reduction of weight....physicians are often handicapped by sharing the common cultural attitude of contempt for fat people and the assumption that all their problems would be solved if they lost weight.

Carole Spitzack
communicologist & author of *Confessing Excess*

Fat people are regarded as ignorant, decadent, stupid, and lazy.

The dynamics of almost all prejudices include a justification for the prejudice based on the laziness of the group being prejudged. Fat people are considered lazy because people practicing bigotry need to believe that fat people are lazy in order to justify their hatred (and discrimination).

Philosopher Paula Rothenberg writes about the ways in which people talk about differences among groups of people even after a particular prejudice is no longer acceptable: "Since race has been obliterated as a category, the only way to explain differences in achievement is by pointing to individual difference. If blacks as a group fail to achieve, the implication is that there is something in their nature that prevents them from achieving. To say they lack a commitment to the Protestant work ethic and a willingness to delay gratification is simply a polite way of restating the old litany that 'Blacks are shiftless and lazy,' but in this more sophisticated form we are left with pointing out a moral deficiency or a deficiency of character which can claim to be colorblind.[6]"

Many will say, of course, that laziness based on race is wrong, but laziness based on body size is obvious. The argument will be made that if fat people were active, they would no longer be fat. The fat itself proves the laziness. But the data suggest otherwise. Active fat people exist, and they don't necessarily lose weight or become thin as they increase their activity.[7]

"What about the children?" The prevailing wisdom is that we have fat kids because we have lazier kids. But a recent longitudinal study found that lean and fat kids were about even in their activity levels, with larger kids actually expending *more* energy.[8] Upon learning that lean kids and fat kids were equally active and were equally consuming energy (food) to match that activity, researchers recommended restricting the diets of fat kids. It apparently never occurred to the researchers that restricting the energy intake of fat kids might lead to the sedentary lifestyle they supposedly deplore.

Such interpretations of the data are grounded in culture more than science. Fat is *obviously* bad, and so if activity alone doesn't *cure obesity,* then "we" have to restrict diet. A vicious circle is set in motion in which kids are punished for being fat by having the fuel that keeps them active and healthy taken from them, leading to sedentary, low-energy lifestyles, confirming the stereotype.

Frances M. Berg, dietitian and author of *Afraid to Eat,* argues that restricting children's diets leads to a number of health and emotional problems. She calls for a health promotion approach that encourages healthy eating and activity for all kids. "The underlying unity of this approach is that what is healthy for the largest kid on the block is also healthy for the thinnest," says Berg. "All children need assurance of acceptance, regardless of size, shape or appearance."

The Doctor's Office

Condescension
drips from his lips.

"You need to take in less calories
than you expend," he says
in slow, elementary tones.

No questions about what I want.

I guess I am just not the one to ask.

All I can think to say is
"'Fewer.'
You mean to say,
'You need to take in *fewer* calories . . .'"

I, of course,
say nothing.

Pattie Thomas
1994

Myth #10: Fat is ugly.

> *I think that at the bottom of the obesity myth in the United States is very much the emotional visceral judgment that being fat is disgusting. That's what is really fueling the obesity myth in America. Since people are socialized, especially in the upper classes, that it is not okay to treat other people as disgusting just because they are different, one has to come up with some rationalization, and the rationalization is that being fat must be horrible for your health.*
>
> Paul Campos
> law professor & author of *The Obesity Myth*

A multi-billion-dollar industry is based upon

the "ideal body." A number of "experts" including physicians, mental health professionals, personal trainers, obesity researchers and diet nutritionists have built their careers and businesses around the desire of people to have the ideal body. These experts are economically dependent on continued acceptance of this impossible standard.

Tabloids follow the weight gains or losses of Anna Nicole Smith, Oprah Winfrey and Elizabeth Taylor with such regularity that one wonders if reporters stake out their bathroom scales. The media coverage of such celebrities, coupled with the reinforcement of thin images on television, in magazines, and throughout advertising, perpetuates this standard and the industry that thrives on it. Shows like *Queer Eye for the Straight Guy, What Not to Wear, Extreme Makeover* and *The Swan* play upon the fascination of audiences with the improvement of "normal" people into the ideal. While fat people are not always the subject of makeovers in these shows or subjected to special criticism when they are, makeovers that are "slimming" are often esteemed. Coupled with the plethora of weight loss products and exercise equipment infomercials that build on the makeover concept, makeovers reinforce the idea of fat bodies being the "before," always needing improvement.

It is no accident that this industry redoubled its efforts at a time when gender stereotypes were being challenged. Naomi Wolf, in her book *The Beauty Myth,* calls this the "beauty backlash." She asserts that the "ideology of beauty is the last one remaining of the old feminine ideologies that still has the power to control those women. . . . [who] would have otherwise [been] relatively uncontrollable."

The myth of ugliness lies in the understanding that beauty is truly in the eye of the beholder. Fat is not inherently ugly because *beauty* is not inherent. Standards of beauty change, with cultures in other places and other times assessing bodies with different measuring sticks. In Western societies between 1400 and 1700, plumpness was a sign of fertility, motherhood, and sexuality. Fat men were regarded as desirable husbands because it indicated their wealth and ability to provide for a family. Psychologist Rita Freedman points out in her book *Beauty Bound* that in the 1800s, "beauty images portrayed matronly plumpness …Doctors encouraged plumpness as a sign of good health (much as doctors are pushing diets a hundred years later.)"

Beauty tastes vary among individuals even within cultures that put a high value on the beauty of certain body types. Thus, fat people *can* be seen as beautiful even in a thin society.

— *Camera Shy* ————————————————————

My husband overheard
her say
the word
"cow."

Was she complimenting
my
bovine eyes
or
my bodacious udders?

I responded by
commenting
LOUDLY
on her
big
butt.

More cat than cow,
I guess.

And you wonder why
I hide BEHIND the
camera.

Pattie Thomas
1994

Looking Good

Five Easy Steps to a Beautiful You

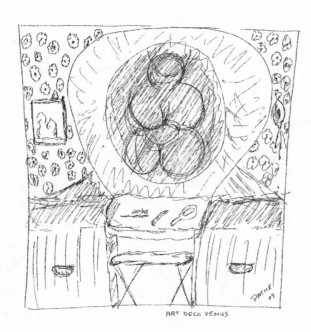

ART DECO VENUS

Don't hate me because I'm beautiful.

L'Oreal Cosmetics Ad

*For once we begin to feel deeply
all the aspects of our lives,
we begin to demand from ourselves
and from our life-pursuits
that they feel in accordance with that joy
which we know ourselves to be capable of.
Our erotic knowledge empowers us,
becomes a lens through which we scrutinize
all aspects of our existence,
forcing us to evaluate those aspects honestly
in terms of their relative meaning
within our lives.*

Audre Lorde

(Haiku Countdown)

Five:
I am not enough
I will never be enough
Insufficient me

Four:
I might be enough
It's a possibility
I have potential

Three:
I'm more than enough
I am more than you can be
I'm above the rest

Two:
I have to be more
I am not allowed to fail
I'm an imposter

One:
Enough is enough
That's enough comparisons
I am who I am

Gently, I remain
Gently, I am becoming
Gently, I am me

Pattie Thomas
2004

Step #1: Make the decision.

> *If the beauty myth is not based on evolution, sex, gender, aesthetics, or God, on what is it based?…The qualities that a given period calls beautiful in women are merely symbols of female behavior that period considers desirable: **The beauty myth is always actually prescribing behavior and not appearance.***

> Naomi Wolf
> feminist & author of *The Beauty Myth*

While teaching a college sociology class, I was explaining the concept of the "white standard" in American society, which is when no mention of white skin is made, while all other skin colors are mentioned explicitly. I challenged my students to take the time to watch television for an evening or read through some popular magazines with an eye for this standard in advertising and fashion. I suggested that even the people of color found in such popular venues are generally lighter-skinned and have more "white" features than their cultural counterparts.

One young white man in the back of the room immediately raised his hand. "Yeah, but isn't that just because that's what people want to see, I mean what people think is beautiful?"

Fighting back tears and the urge to scream at him, I responded that beauty is created by culturally based beliefs, with different cultures at different times defining beauty in different ways. Then, no longer able to hold back my frustration and pain in front of a class of 70 people, most of whom were half my age, I said, "I think it is sad that our society has made it so that so few of us can be considered beautiful. Surely we want to enjoy life more than that."

I almost didn't recover. A small voice in the back of my brain screamed, *"Now you did it! Way to go with the defensive posture. Way to go, Fatso!"* Years of silencing told me that a woman such as me, a fat woman, was not supposed to speak of beauty, at least not unless it was connected to a goal of weight loss or admiring a thin woman.

The student's question was an important one, even if it was not based on an accurate or sensitive treatment of the subject of beauty. Any discussion of beauty invariably leads to the always present: "So what? Aren't we just talking about personal preferences? How can we change a person's tastes? Why should we try?"

The answer by feminists and cultural critics is usually medically based, stating that narrow standards of preferred body types lead to the high prevalence of eating disorders and the terrible consequences of radical dieting and extensive exercising. I'd like to suggest that this response offers little room for a full understanding of beauty, and leaves us in the position of confirming the medicalization of bodies.

The medical answer steps around the question of taste and suggests a moral or political claim that someone is "just wrong" for liking what they like because it causes harm. I don't like answers that draw lines in the sand without offering a way out for those who are seeking a path. The "it's just wrong" answer never leaves a way out for a seeker.

I am not arguing that the pain of distorted eating and exercising behaviors is not real, or that people who benefit from therapies aimed at dealing with eating disorders are somehow responsible for perpetuating the oppression of female *and* male bodies. Nor am I suggesting that narrow standards of beauty have no part in the development of distorted eating and exercising behaviors. Narrow standards of beauty do cause harm, and are clearly in need of examination. But more than medical arguments are available to confront the damage, and these arguments need to be raised.

These standards of beauty hurt everyone, because they make the vast majority of us feel unworthy, not good enough. Such pain is not a disorder; it is extremely orderly. It is a reasonable response to oppression.

Distorted eating and exercising behaviors are but a symptom of a far more pervasive problem, and that problem is not psychological or medical. It is social. If the only stated opposition to what Kim Chernin, in her book *The Obsession,* called the "tyranny of slenderness" is one that calls for the prevention of eating disorders, then we are in danger of reifying the very system that needs to be changed.

But where should the discussion begin if not with eating disorders, drastic dieting or self-esteem issues among young women? It begins in global post-industrial capitalism. It begins with an understanding of consumption, and the part consumption plays in the everyday lives of citizens in consumption-oriented economies.

This is a place that many fat people dread, because the rhetoric among those who critique consumption almost always includes the fat American as a symbol of consumption. This usage of fatness needs to be confronted because it is a naïve analysis of consumption and the consequences of consumption. It needs to be confronted because blaming fat people for the problems of over-consumption falls prey to the very mechanism that sets up over-consumption—the belief that we cannot be satisfied with who we are, and that our only hope is to buy more things in an effort to be who we are *supposed* to be.

It is virtually impossible in today's market to separate the concept of health from the concept of beauty. Many products often list as benefits both looking better and becoming healthier. The words "health and beauty" roll off the tongue as easily as "bread and butter," "his and hers" and "sex and violence."

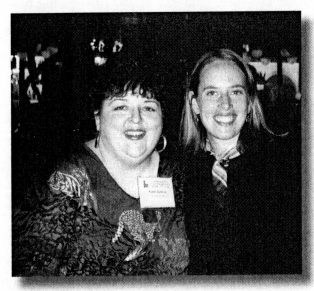

1998. San Francisco American Sociological Association & Sociologists for Women in Society conventions. Hanging out with Boston College grad student Julie Childers, schmoozing and having fun.

Most of us never give much thought to what we are being told through the pairing of the word "health" with the word "beauty." People see others who *look good* and assume that they are healthy. People see others who lack style and wonder about their health.

As a fat person, I wish I had a dime for every time someone has expressed concern for my health because of my weight. A typical conversation goes something like this:

"Pattie, are you losing weight?"

"Not that I know about. I don't weigh myself. I don't consider my weight my business. I take care of my body as well as I can, and I let my body weight be whatever it is."

"Yeah, it's good that you exercise. But, well, what about your heart or diabetes?"

"My heart and blood sugar level are fine, thank you. Exercise is good for those things."

At this point, I get annoyed because the person is requiring a medical history from me, and usually I change the subject. However, many times the person insists on giving me his or her own diet and weight loss history. Often they tell me about a cousin or niece who has had weight loss surgery and plastic surgery. Invariably, they mention how much better the person looks now that they have lost weight.

I usually don't encourage such conversations. I often just listen politely, try to change the subject, or I say something direct, like "I really hate the way that Wilson woman never tells young people about the extensive plastic surgery she's had to have to look normal after her weight loss surgery," and they stop talking to me about it.

Sometimes, however, when the weight loss surgery topic arises and I hear about how good the person looks, I ask about health since the surgery. Often, I am told that the person isn't really doing that well. They are still dealing with life after surgery. This is usually told in such a way that the sacrifice seems worth it because the person is able to go places and looks so much better.

It is rare that the conversation is reversed and the good health of the relative is mentioned *before* the good looks. The words "they look good" are considered sufficient to justify the surgery or weight loss plan. In other words, whatever pain or ill health has resulted from the surgery has been worth it because the person "looks so much better" thin. Health and beauty remain inseparable.

Such a priority of looks over health is not limited to street conversations.

The first time a doctor offered the weight loss surgery option to me was about a year before I became ill with lupus. In the previous six years I had faced and overcome a number of health problems. I had survived addiction to the prescription drugs I used for nearly two years, both diet pills to lose weight and the Valium that I used to sleep at night. I survived giving birth to a premature, stillborn son, which had left my body and my emotional state weary and stressed, to put it mildly. More recently, I had had a melanoma lesion removed and a hysterectomy prompted by several years of positive Pap smears. Both procedures had been done in time, and I was cancer free.

I was riding a bike and walking to and from school. I was taking a weight-training class. I wasn't particularly happy in my own skin, but I was beginning to feel good again. I was a survivor in several senses of that word, and I was rebuilding my life and my health.

My physician was aware of my history, and knew that I was getting healthier. So when I arrived for a follow-up visit, I was blindsided when she hit me with the "you need to lose weight" talk. She had pamphlets about weight loss surgery and a referral in mind.

She sat me down in her office and said the bouts with cancer were "typical" with someone who was "morbidly" obese. I said I wasn't so sure about that. "Don't you have patients who are thin but have had dysplasia and/or melanomas?" She admitted that to be true. Then she said, and I remember her words almost exactly:

"Pattie, you're an obviously brilliant woman. You are poised and articulate. It seems like every part of your life is going well right now except your weight. You obviously have lots of self-discipline, and I believe you have truly tried to lose weight. I would hate to think that all that would go to waste because all people could see is how fat you are. You are in good health except for your weight. You are the perfect candidate for weight loss surgery. I'd like for you to consider it. You could be a beautiful woman who could have it all."

I find this conversation to be one of the most vivid examples in my personal life of the doublespeak that goes on regarding weight loss. After surviving a miscarriage, drug addiction, surgery and two potential cancers, my physician could not leave well enough alone. I had overcome so much medically and had come out the other side fairly healthy. By her own admission, the only thing that was "wrong" was that my body did not conform to a preconceived image.

I did not have heart disease, high cholesterol, high blood pressure, or diabetes. I had neither gained nor lost a significant amount of weight in the past year. I was stable, healthier than I had been in years, and had settled into my graduate degree program nicely. Rather than congratulating me for surviving a great deal of stressors and some close calls medically and then telling me to come back for a checkup in a year, My physician decided that I was the "perfect candidate" for further trauma in the guise of weight loss surgery.

Weight loss surgery was supposed to be a last resort for "obese" people whose health is failing. That is why the doctor began the conversation by suggesting the close calls with cancer were connected to "morbid obesity." The fact that she backed off on the point when I confronted her does not mean that it was not part of her logic in

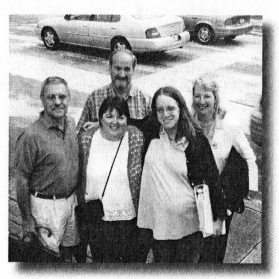

Celebrating becoming a doctor, age 44.

left to right:
Dr. Jay Gubrium,
dissertation chair;
Dr. Pattie Thomas
(for about 1 hour),
Mike Ryan, Erica Owens,
Dr. Connie Sheehan.

Photo 2001 Carl Wilkerson

recommending the surgery.

In this scenario, "morbid obesity" is both the premise and the conclusion. My physician was assigning me to an "at risk" group and then tried to argue that because I was in that group, the assignation was an appropriate one. I was supposed to accept as a given that my obesity meant I was at risk for serious illnesses (morbidity), and I was simultaneously supposed to accept that because I was at risk, it proved that my obesity was of the type that merited surgery.

The original assignation (morbidly obese) was done **axiomatically.** I was morbidly obese because I weighed over a certain number. The proposition that "being fat is bad" is made without much empirical study to support the claim. It's an **axiomatic statement,** made on a the basis of a self-evident truth rather than research.

Most studies on "obesity" are done with the assumption that losing weight is a goal worthy of achievement, and are not based in empirical understandings of fat bodies. The truth-value of the statement "fat is bad" comes from an axiom, not from any empirical data or any other rigorous observations.

In the 1920s, a number of middle class women wanted to be fashionable "flappers" and wanted their doctors to provide the potions or methodologies to make them slimmer. The medicalization of fat was derived from their cultural belief that being fat was bad and thin was "in." As doctors provided these women with "treatments" to lose weight, they began to look for medical reasons for the "condition" for which they were "treating" them.

From the beginning, such "obesity research" was about weight loss, not about understanding fat bodies. No one asked, much less studied, the question: "Is being fat bad?" The research conducted then—and, usually, now—merely searches for ways that fat can be considered bad, and assumes that all fat people are the same and, in fact, that all people are potentially fat people.

Once one ceases to examine the *truth* of an axiom, the object of study merely *assumes* the axiom. All questions of study come from the axiom.

Once researchers made "fat is bad" axiomatic, the possibility

Co-hosting / co-producing
First Person, Plural
2002-2004

Photo 2001 Stephen Thomas

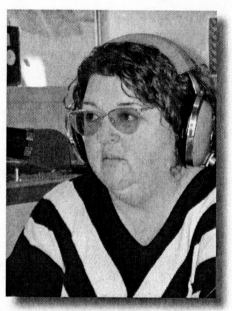

of testing the proposition for truth within their axiomatic framework became impossible. They would have to unfix it as an axiom. They would have to take the axiom out of the set of first principles. All axiomatic models are about establishing the set of principles that are true and then deriving arguments and proofs from those fixed principles.

In the "fat is bad" model, anyone who weighs more than a pre-designated amount is a "perfect candidate" for weight loss "treatment," regardless of the state of their health. In fact, weighing more than the pre-designated amount is the only way "morbid obesity" is defined.

I was not in ill health because of some symptom or indicator my physician observed medically. I was simply fat ("obese") and therefore in danger of illness (morbidity). Fatness was and is the only factor under consideration.

The reasoning is circular. The premise is that I am at risk because of my weight, and the conclusion is that the fact that I am at risk demonstrates that the assumed relationship between my weight and the risk is valid in my case. My being at risk both was proven by my having a body type defined by its need for surgery, and proved my need for surgery.

In this model and reasoning, if a fat person is in bad health, she or he should risk the surgery because she or he is in bad health and the surgery (losing weight) may help. If a fat person is in good health, this model and reasoning assumes she or he should risk the surgery because "everyone knows" that without weight loss, she or he will eventually be in bad health and it is better to do the surgery when one is healthy and can handle it better.

If there is no distinguishing between fat people who are healthy and fat people who are not healthy before they have the surgery, then on what basis can one judge the outcome of the surgery?

Weight is the only indicator of health in this scenario. The physician is saying that all people weighing more than a specified amount should have the surgery in order to ensure their good health. How does one know that a fat person has bad health? Because he or she is fat. How does one know that a fat person has good health? Because he or she loses weight.

If one is healthy going into weight loss surgery, there is no other way besides weight loss to judge the outcome of the surgery. Continued good health cannot be ascribed to the surgery. One can only argue about what might have happened if the surgery had not taken place.

If the surgery leads to ill health, as it frequently does, the physician or surgeon is then free to argue that the "morbid obesity" and not the surgery caused the ill health. This way of thinking often justifies the surgeon writing "obesity" as cause of death when a "perfect candidate" dies from complications from weight loss surgery.

One might argue that weight loss surgery could be considered preventative. Surgery, however, is a pretty drastic treatment for

Coming from good people with good genes ... ————

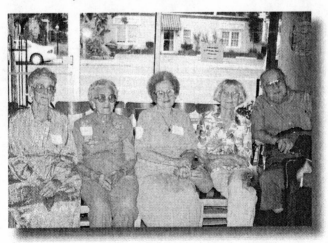

My great-aunts and -uncle, all in their 80s and 90s.

Photo 1999
Pattie Thomas

prevention. Preventative surgery is only called for in situations where it is *assured* that the condition the treatment is preventing almost always leads to ill health.

The whole medical argument for extreme weight loss methods supposedly rests on the assertion that a correlation exists between being fat and poor health and/or early death. Even if this were an overall trend, the general case would be superseded by individual cases.

One wouldn't treat *all* African Americans for sickle cell anemia because sickle cell anemia is prevalent in African Americans. Consider the implications of physicians who would avoid making careful examinations and diagnoses of the individual patient before prescribing treatment, basing recommendations simply on a patient's membership in various groups and the patient's other observed levels of various factors without regard for individualized considerations. At that point, why even have a human doctor? One could feed demographic information into a computer that could spit out a treatment plan without even examining an individual. Private companies that train local police departments in the mechanics of racial profiling would be pleased to discover the potential of this new application of their products: medical profiling.

The whole point of a doctor-patient encounter is to allow for individual variations that make patient-specific treatment important.

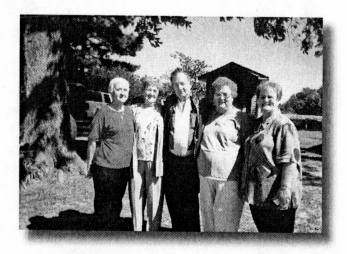

My mom (second from right), aunts and uncle, all in their 60s and 70s.

Photo 1999
Pattie Thomas

A plethora of conditions besides risk factors may be present to help the physician determine a course of action. While some treatments may be established as appropriate in the "average" case, often it is true that individuals have mitigating circumstances that make applicability of a certain diagnosis or treatment inappropriate. For example, the presence of conditions that may cause sudden weight loss such as cancers or ulcers gives patients with some extra fat an edge over thinner patients.

In addition to factors that the physician can observe or assess, simply listening to patients' impressions and experiences of their own bodies can provide important information to the physician that is not available through direct measurements. Weight should be one small indicator in this host of factors. Treating weight as a primary factor may be an easy way for a physician to assess health, but it is not a responsible way to do so.

I was in good health. I was fat. Being in good health was seen as a reason to proceed with a drastic "treatment."

I can't imagine anybody accepting such a twisted deal from a physician. "I've looked over your chart. You're in perfect health. We'd better schedule you for surgery just in case something bad happens."

There may be cases where surgery is advisable in order to prevent further disease development. Certainly, my hysterectomy after six years of positive Pap smears was done in part as a prevention of cervical cancer. But no physician should advise a hysterectomy just because a patient is a sexually active woman, "just in case." (Being female, by the way, has a higher correlation to cervical cancer than being fat has to any disease or disorder.)

However, my doctor did not make a *medical* argument for my weight loss. Her reasoning depended on a concept of beauty, not a concept of health. If health was the concern, then why push for drastic weight loss measurements for an otherwise healthy person?

I had been advised to have the hysterectomy because cancer cells were already in my body and were on the verge of becoming invasive. Only after a number of other treatments that failed to completely get rid of the cells did my doctor recommend surgery, and I was told to get another opinion before making a final decision. No such caution was advised with the proposed weight loss surgery.

In the end, however, my physician's argument did not rest on previous or future illnesses. Health wasn't really the concern. Her concern was that none of my personal accomplishments, skills or character would be acceptable in a fat body. All the good things in my life would "go to waste" because of the prejudices of others.

Imagine this conversation happening with someone from a stigmatized religious or ethnic background: "Make sure people don't know about your religious upbringing or your ethnic background because all the good things about you will go to waste if they find out what you are. Look, I know a guy who can make you look more 'white.' No one will ever have to know who you really are."

Of course, unscrupulous doctors have made such proposals in back-alley clinics. But this was a modern day medical office at the end of the 20th century. The doctor was essentially telling me that she had technology for me to be able to pass for thin. She was advising that whatever risks cutting my body open would create to my health and well-being, the surgery would be worth it because otherwise, the prejudice of others would make my assets go to waste.

To a more cynical eye, such encounters seem a perfect way to generate more business for physicians. It was not enough that I should be healthy. I was a regular customer for a couple of years, and now I was in danger of not needing medical attention. I will concede that in my specific case, my doctor was probably acting out of compassion and trying to use a "holistic" approach. But the general case is exactly what the cynic would suggest.

Medicalization of fat allows physicians to make more money and treat more patients. It expands medical power and increases medical intrusion into our bodies. It is finding sickness where none exists so the medical establishment can have a bigger market.

I took the weight loss surgery literature home. I didn't feel right about it, though. Something about the whole thing gnawed at me. For one thing, the pamphlet stated that 30 percent of the people who had this surgery had serious complications. This was a pamphlet *promoting* the surgery—the propaganda on which they put the most positive face they could.

I just couldn't see it. I couldn't get past that 30 percent.

I had just had a hysterectomy after being told every time I was given a progressively more invasive treatment for the condition that there was only a 1 percent chance that the latest treatment would not clear up the condition. Every time, my condition got worse after the treatment, not better. I kept landing right in that supposed 1 percent. So why would I take a chance on 30 percent?

To add insult to injury, I spoke about the surgery with the therapist I was seeing at the time, a woman who was fat herself, a woman who had not been able to lose weight despite considerable efforts to do so. Instead of helping me sort through the statistics, she suggested that I was quite lucky to have such a caring doctor and insurance that would cover the surgery. Some of her other clients wanted the surgery and couldn't get it. Maybe this was a godsend.

As with the physician, the therapist was making what amounted to an argument about beauty rather than health. I can almost imagine a conversation in a women's restroom at a dance club:

"Did you hear that Pattie's doctor is going to recommend she gets one of those gastric bypass surgeries?"

"I wish I could do that. I'm just not fat enough, I guess. I heard there was a doctor who would write a recommendation if you were just 50 pounds overweight. I'm not sure my parents' insurance would cover it, though. I wonder if they have enough money to pay for it out of pocket."

"Oh, Pattie is *soooo* lucky. Her doctor said 'yes,' and her insurance will cover it. She's going to be *soooo* pretty."

"Yeah, but I hear Pattie doesn't want to do the surgery. She just doesn't appreciate how lucky she is."

The "everybody's doing it" argument seems rather juvenile on the surface, but a great deal of pressure is put on fat people, and fat women especially, to conform. The supposed health considerations of weight loss hide an agenda of conformity that ensures that people do not deviate from norms too far.

As Wolf suggests in the quote earlier in this section, beauty, and the weight loss one supposedly has to create in order to be beautiful, is more about acceptable behaviors than it is about a concept of beauty, or, for that matter, a concept of health. My therapist was, in effect, telling me that I was lucky to have a chance to conform to society's standards of beauty and to have health care coverage that would pay for the process.

Inherent in the "everybody's doing it" argument is the underlying competition women often create with each other.

Feminists often shy away from the topic of female competition, but women know it exists. We know that many of us compare ourselves to other women, assessing our femininity and acceptability on the basis of how well we compete with those other women. The shape of our bodies is certainly a large part of that comparison process.

Fatness in this competition is regarded as a major axis upon which femininity can be judged. If you want to be catty about a particular person, you merely say to a friend, "My, doesn't she look fat?" or "Wow, she's really put on weight."

This happens even among fat women. I decided after suffering from pneumonia in 2002 that I was going to strengthen my body. I found a relatively inexpensive aqua therapy program that allowed me to slowly regain strength. I went in to the program with the understanding that I would never be weighed and that weight loss would never be my goal. There were others in the program who were trying to lose weight, but I was never pressured, and my goals of gaining strength, flexibility, stamina and balance were fully supported. It was an environment in which I felt safe and encouraged.

Another woman in the program came on one of my regular days. She was a fat woman, only slightly smaller than I am. She wore beautiful swimsuits and had obviously found a great place for larger women's clothes. One day, when we were getting ready to go into the pool to work out, I complimented her on the suit she was wearing.

"Thank you," she said.

"Where do you find your suits?" I asked.

"Well, I get them at a store in the mall, but I wear the largest size they have." Then, in a very catty tone, "I don't think they'd have a suit that would fit *you*."

I smiled back and wished her a happy workout, walking away feeling ambushed, but there was more to come. While I was in the pool, she came up beside me and whispered, "You should really buy a suit with a skirt. They will hide your thighs and make you look slimmer."

Suddenly my sanctuary was violated. The pool that I had grown to love was a place of competition and catty conversations. I told her that I bought my swimsuit for utility, not style, politely thanked her for her concern, and then I swam to another part of the pool as quickly as I could. I was so shaken by the encounter that I left early, unable to finish my workout for the day.

I decided to avoid this woman in the future, and had the flexibility of schedule to do so. I resolved to confront her the next time and to speak with the trainer if she persisted, but was pleased when "the next time" didn't happen.

Such competition is not limited, of course, to female cat fights. People compete with each other in all sorts of arenas, including business, market places, schools and sports. Fatness is often used rhetorically to distinguish a winner from a loser. In fact, "big fat loser" is a well-known epithet at many sporting events.

Pointing out my fatness was one way some of my fellow graduate students used to assert their superiority over me in a highly competitive department. This was done both behind my back and to my face, with both ill and good intentions.

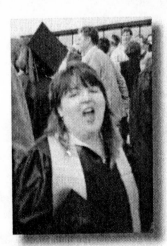

One fellow student confided in me, after getting to know me better, that he was surprised to find out how smart I was. Some of the other students had told him

Graduating with a B.A. from the University of South Florida in 1995.

Photo 1995 Carl Wilkerson

about me before he met me, saying "her ass is big enough to set a table on," and concluding that I was obviously "unstable."

Another friend begged me to never use a cane or mention lupus when talking to potential employers, because "you already have the weight thing working against you."

One wonders if graduate school was less competitive, would such assessments and assigning of stigmas be evoked?

Bigotry comes not only from stereotypes and unintentional repeating of cultural ideas about groups of people. Bigotry also comes from allowing certain strategies used by those who compete to be successful strategies.

Stigmatization isn't always done "unthinkingly." It can be a part of deliberate competitive activity, as well. If your chief competitor is leaning on you too hard, attaching a stigma to her or him can slow her or him down quite a bit. Describing others as fat, or, more accurately, fatter, is a convenient and efficient way of asserting superiority in a highly competitive situation.

Suppose two parties are in competition for a contract. Their bids are similar in content and cost. In the course of an interview, the first bidder tells the contractor that the second bidder is fat. The contractor then chooses the first bidder over the second solely on the basis of the description. This strategy works because the bigoted description separated the first bidder from the second. However, the key element was *the reaction of the contractor.*

"Fatness" evoked a set of assumptions about the second bidder that was only meaningful if both the first bidder and the contractor understand that set of assumptions. That set of assumptions gives the first bidder an edge. If the contractor didn't share—or endorse—the first bidder's assumptions, the competitive strategy would not work.

One of the reasons some people no longer refer to African Americans with the "n-word" is that nowadays using the word hurts their chances in competition more than raises them. This kind of bigotry is not about beliefs, but about exploiting beliefs for personal gain in competitions.

My therapist, and even my physician, may have been concerned about my ability to compete in a world of bigots. Perhaps, however, their personal reactions were based in their *own* fears and strategies in a competitive culture that pits woman against woman, professional against professional, and intelligence against intelligence.

The timing of the advised treatment was interesting. I had been defined as "morbidly obese" for a number of years by that point, but had never before been advised to consider weight loss surgery, even when I was having specific health problems. What *was* happening in my life at the point when weight loss surgery was encouraged was that I was finishing my Ph.D. and moving toward becoming a professional woman.

Before, I was either "working class" or "student." The "concern" of these professional women may have been rooted in the competition many professional women feel with other women of their class, even those in different fields, rather than genuine regard for my well-being.

The relationship between health care professional and client is a power relationship even in the best of circumstances. Using bigotry to convince a client or patient to undergo treatments that offer monetary rewards for the health care worker helps keep the fat client or patient under the professional's control. Thus, bigoted language enhances the competitive edge of the health care professional by ensuring that the object of bigotry will continue to be a client or patient.

Health care professionals are often given *carte blanche* to use any means possible to convince clients or patients the advice they give is worthwhile. Their status allows them to justify their advice by virtue of *who they are* as much as by what they say. Thus, using bigoted language as a resource to motivate the client or patient is often not regarded as being bigoted due to their status.

On a number of occasions I have been the only sociologist at a table of scholars discussing health care treatment for older adults. The medical model, which is often held not only by physicians, but also by nurses, psychologists, physical therapists and other health care professionals, suggests that treatment should be oriented either to a specific disease state or, at least, a specific patient. When I suggest that attention should be given to the social context of treatment, most of these professionals believe that means the individual should be taught how to cope with whatever social factors contribute to the patient's health or ill health. Suggesting that the focus should be on those people or ideas in society that are creating the social factors is often met with a resounding, "Oh well, we can't do much about that, can we? People are going to think what they are going to think."

I suspect that critiquing the cultural and social pressures that would lead a health care professional to suggest a healthy person undergo major surgery in order to look better and be more acceptable to others was beyond the scope of my therapist. Both the physician and the therapist were viewing my situation with a narrow view of what was good for a patient, a view that would lead to less stigmatization, but not necessarily more health.

I also suspect there was a sense that I should not even question the doctor's advice. My therapist may have believed she was not qualified to question the doctor's premise that fat people should be treated even if they are healthy. She may have seen it as her job to support the medical authority by getting me to accept the doctor's advice. In that kind of quest, convention allows for health care workers to use whatever arguments are available to help break down the so-called denial of the patient.

She may have been offering the "everybody's doing it" and "aren't you so lucky" arguments as means of helping me overcome my fear of being cut open. She may have even seen my hesitation as phobic or rebellious.

Fat people who remain fat are often treated by psychologists as rebellious, holding on to their fat selves as a "cushion" or "padding" between the "real" thin self and the world.

Medical and nursing journals are filled with articles about patient compliance. Most of these articles regard patients as rebellious or ignorant in their refusal to follow doctor's orders. In response to such patients, health care professionals are taught a number of strategies.

Many articles encourage education. As a fat person, I cannot tell you the number of pamphlets I've been handed to educate me about calories, exercise and weight loss.

I would guess that most fat people are as amused as I have been when the physician or nurse comes in the room and says, "Now you may not know this, but being overweight is related to a number of health conditions."

We know. We hear it all the time. In fact, we probably know more about nutrition or, at least, the nutritional value of food than most health care professionals. Any person who spent 30 years dieting has probably memorized all sorts of details about food, calorie expenditures and body fat.

Another strategy is to identify the motivation of a patient. This strategy suggests that the lack of patient compliance is due to lack of motivation or lack of being *properly* motivated.

I think this might be what my doctor and my therapist were trying to do by using beauty arguments. Both women may have decided that I just wasn't motivated by health considerations, or I would have been successful in previous attempts. I needed to understand all the advantages of this procedure in order to comply with doctor's orders.

In the strategy of motivation, a lie might be as good as the truth, and one motive is as good as the next, as long as the patient complies.

The saddest part of the whole encounter with my therapist for me, as I look back on it, is the extent to which I believe she was incapable of helping me sort through the details because she had her own body issues.

I once saw a counselor several years previously who, in the course of the intake interview, told me that I obviously had problems with my mother. This statement by someone who had known me about 10 minutes was not only premature, but clearly motivated by something else. I know this because the counselor's pronouncement was followed by about 10 minutes of her telling me all the problems she had with *her* mother.

After about 35 minutes of this ridiculous interview I stood up, thanked her very much for her time, told her that I hoped she and her mother worked things out, and then I left.

I should have realized that my therapist was dealing with *her* issues about being fat more than my issues. Her advice regarding the weight loss surgery was a non sequitor in her mostly hands-off approach to therapy. She rarely told me what to do or even suggested outcomes, opting, usually, to let me talk myself into something.

Looking back, it was quite obvious that she had issues and that her issues were coloring her advice. Unfortunately, it took me about six months after the weight loss surgery talk to come to that realization.

In spite of this advice, or, rather, because of it, I decided weight loss surgery was not for me. I was fully vindicated about a year later when I saw an episode of *60 Minutes* that investigated a weight loss surgeon in my home town who had lost patients on the operating table at a rate of nine times the national average. It turns out he had left one state for malpractice and had set up shop in my home state without telling anyone about his previous record.

I couldn't believe my eyes when his name appeared on my television screen. It was the doctor to whom I had been referred. Listening to my gut (and keeping it) had probably saved my life.

The weight loss surgery discussion with my physician was not an unusual conversation in my life. Since about the age of 11, I've had "the weight loss discussion" with my doctors. Throughout my teens and 20s, the discussion usually went like this:

"All of your blood work is normal. Your blood pressure is a little

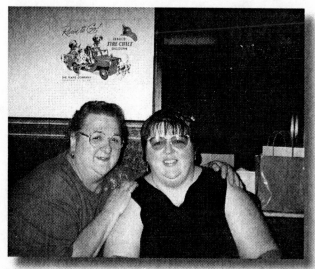

2002.
Mom
(LaVelle Thomas)
came for a visit
to Victoria,
British Columbia,
where Carl and I
moved after
I graduated
with the Ph.D.

Photo 2002
Stephen Thomas

low. You have a few allergy symptoms, but nothing a dose of antihistamine can't handle. You would be in superb health if you lost weight. Here's a low-calorie diet. Make sure you do a little exercise every day. You know being overweight is bad for you. Come back and see me in six months for a checkup and try to lose 20 pounds by then."

One doctor actually said to me after a full physical, "You certainly are a healthy, fat dear."

Don't get me wrong. For most of the time I took the doctors' advice seriously. I worried about my health and I tried to lose weight. I was always on some "plan" or another. My weight yo-yoed quite a bit, always ending the cycle with a body larger than it was at the beginning of the last attempt to lose weight.

I felt like a failure most of the time. I spent literal years of my life counting something about my food or activity. I could name the nutritional content of practically any food product on the market. I read labels constantly. I drank all sorts of concoctions. I spent thousands of dollars. I lost hundreds of pounds.

The only good thing I did for myself through all of this was exercise. But I never felt good about exercising because it was never enough

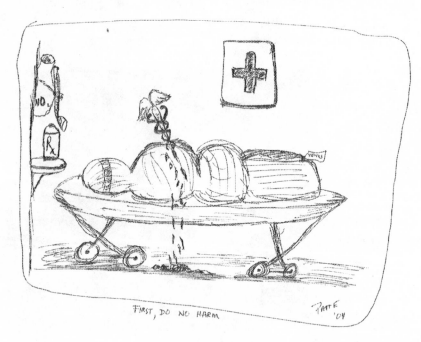

FIRST, DO NO HARM

PATTE '04

to lose "all the weight."

All of this started at the age of 11, and it colored my life completely.

At the age of 29, after quitting a job I hated, I became depressed and practically agoraphobic. I literally went weeks without leaving my apartment or even getting out of my pajamas.

When I did go out, I was scared of people. I made runs to the grocery store for food and liquor in the middle of the night to avoid seeing people. I ate a lot. I drank a lot. I cried a lot. I watched a lot of soap operas.

My marriage was falling apart. My life felt worthless. I had no job and no energy to find a job. I was convinced that I was not worth a damn and that I had failed in every way a person could fail.

After about four months of this complete breakdown, my husband at the time contacted a psychotherapist, and I began to see her. Now the only time I left the apartment was for midnight runs to the grocery store and seeing the therapist every two weeks.

She put me on an antidepressant. She listened to me. She helped me see how trapped I was in my marriage (a weird, ironic twist, since my husband had found her). She helped me gain the strength to find a low-stress job that got me out of the house. She helped me understand how my being raped at the age of five had shaped my life and my choices.

She also told me that being fat was my way of coping with all of this stress.

After a few months of therapy, I got "serious" about weight loss. I wanted to be beautiful. I wanted to look and feel beautiful. I went to a bariatric clinic. "Bariatrics" is the branch of medicine devoted to "treating" obesity.

The clinic had a group approach that involved a weekly meeting with other patients at the clinic. We talked about food as if we were addicts. We discussed "trigger" foods. We kept extensive diaries of what we ate, what we felt when we ate, and a list of measurements of body dimensions and weight. We were also given a daily dose of synthetic speed to curb our appetites and a weekly shot of B-12 to "restore our energy."

Between the psychotherapy and the bariatric clinic, I thought I was finally taking care of myself. I was on a 600- to 800-calorie-a-day diet. I often went an entire day without eating. I walked and eventually ran two miles a day.

I lost weight, a lot of weight. I was happy. I was sexy. I was competent. I thought I had finally solved the riddle.

After moving away from the town where the clinic and the psychotherapist were, I found a new doctor who continued the prescriptions. He weighed me weekly and gave me B-12 shots. He called me "the amazing shrinking woman" and said he bragged about me to other patients. I was an inspiration.

I landed the best job I'd ever had. I was going to be okay.

But I started having trouble sleeping at night. My menstrual cycle started getting wacky. A gynecologist gave me Valium for severe cramps. I found Valium counteracted the effects of the speed and let me sleep. I talked the regular physician into giving me Valium prescriptions as well; I had to increase the dose.

I had two doctors and two pharmacies, allowing me to get twice as much Valium as prescribed. In addition, I found drinking light beer satisfied me more than food. I frequently had days where I didn't eat and had 600 calories of beer. Calorie counting was probably the only thing that kept me from being constantly drunk. I kept running two to four miles a day.

I didn't seek out a psychotherapist in my new town, but my husband and I did start seeing a marriage counselor. The thinner I got, the more confident I got about leaving my husband. Eventually, I did just that.

I was 31 years old, I was the thinnest I had been in my adult life, I was single again, and I had the best job I had ever had.

But as good as things looked on the outside, they were crazy on the inside. I was an imposter, and I needed speed and Valium and alcohol to keep up the act. As it turned out, it was not a sustainable strategy.

In August of 1988 I had a nervous breakdown and ended up in an inpatient codependency program. There I was told I was an "addict." I didn't admit to the Valium use, but I was told I needed to get off the speed. I had begun abusing laxatives as well, and was told I was a "borderline bulimic."

I quit alcohol, speed and Valium cold turkey with only a daily self-help meeting for support. My keeping the Valium a secret could have killed me. I quit cold a six-month habit of daily Valium use. I was wide-awake for three solid weeks. I was so tired from not sleeping that I made big mistakes at work and was in danger of losing my job. I was extremely lucky that my heart didn't stop beating from the stress. I found out only later than it is best to taper off Valium a little at a time.

My first year without drugs and alcohol was one of the most stressful years of my life. I finalized my divorce. I got pregnant by a man I barely knew and had only slept with twice. When I was 16

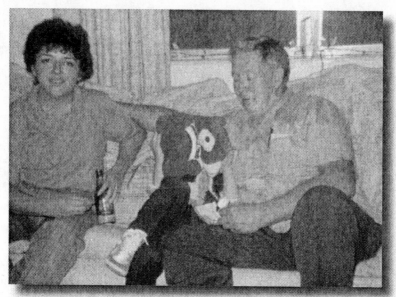

Photo 1987 LaVelle Thomas

Notice the beer in my hand. That's me with my niece and my dad in 1987 after losing 130 pounds using speed, Valium, and drinking nothing but light beer. Most people believed I was happy. I felt like an imposter all the time. I was afraid I was going to gain weight or die trying not to gain.

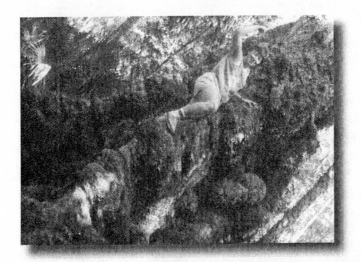

By 1989, on my 32nd birthday, I was off the pills and trying to get my life back together. However, I used these photos for years as motivation to lose weight as I continued to regain the weight I had lost on the pills.

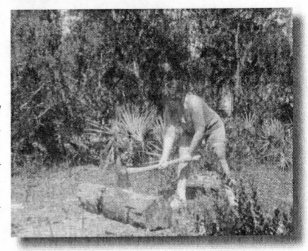

weeks pregnant, my water broke. The baby's heart stopped beating. The physician decided to induce labor, and I had a stillborn son.

I concentrated on work to deal with the pain of loss. After working very hard to regain the respect of my colleagues, I was laid off from my wonderful job when the company downsized. I filed for bankruptcy.

By my 33rd birthday I was emotionally, physically and spiritually drained. I decided that in order to regain control of my life, I needed to lose the weight I had regained after stopping the diet pills and becoming pregnant. I joined Overeaters Anonymous.

I had overcome drug addiction and alcohol. I told myself that the last problem I had to conquer was my "eating addiction." I was a hard case, I told myself, so I joined a branch of OA called "OA-HOW." I came to call this group by a nickname I heard: "the Food Nazis."

I had a sponsor to whom I "surrendered" my eating habits. She told me what to eat, and I would eat that and nothing else. The diet was a high-protein, low-carbohydrate diet. At meetings we not only weighed in, we announced our weight to the group and were given a round of applause for any weight loss. Weight gain required us to describe "what went wrong" during the past week. Meetings were quite ritualized.

After a loss of 65 pounds in a little less than three months (almost all of the weight I had gained after getting off the diet pills), I got very ill. It turned out that my kidneys were starting to shut down from the diet I was on. I was told that if I didn't start eating vegetables and fruits and drinking a great deal of water, I would be put in a hospital.

I quit OA-HOW because my sponsor told me the nurse was wrong in telling me I needed to eat more, and that I was just looking for a way to justify my addiction.

I spent the summer sick with asthma and pneumonia. I gained 80 pounds in the next six months.

I didn't give up dieting, but I did give up radical diets. I was now going to learn how to "eat sensibly."

But something had changed. I couldn't lose any weight on a 1,500-calorie-a-day diet. I was strict and didn't gain any weight, but I didn't lose, either.

I again filled notebooks with lists of the food I had eaten and my body measurements. I kept logs about my exercising. My whole life could be summed up in energy consumption and expenditures. But I just couldn't lose weight.

Fortunately, it was during this time that I was introduced to women's studies and, in particular, to issues about women and health.

I had read *Fat is a Feminist Issue* by Susie Orbach several years before, but the book had simply convinced me I was fat because I had "issues" that needed to be "resolved."

I had some naïve understanding of women's issues, but I had always regarded feminism as something irrelevant to a working class woman. I did not envy my father's or my uncle's jobs. They worked dirty, physical jobs that didn't always cover the family expenses. My grandmothers, my aunts and my mother had always done some form of work outside the home such as laundry, ironing, babysitting for neighbors, factory shifts or home-based businesses. These were jobs that supplemented their husbands' incomes and helped make the family's ends meet.

I had a business college degree and worked in corporate offices. I didn't make as much money as my father had as a mechanic, but I certainly had better working conditions. The rhetoric of equal pay seemed irrelevant, and the equal pay issue was the only feminist issue I knew.

Women's studies changed that. I learned a lot about how race and class intertwined with gender to limit the life chances of many people. I learned that questions of sexuality and beauty needed to be explored in light of a long history of exploitation of a number of people, both women and men.

I was lucky enough during this time to see a feminist therapist who helped me see my "emotional" problems in light of the public issues that gave my life context. I stopped thinking of *my* being the problem and started thinking about the limitations systems of power placed on my life chances. This new knowledge empowered me. I began to question everything I had been told about life. I mean *everything.*

"Everything" included fatness.

My first hint that fatness might not be as clearcut as I once thought was when I read the following in *The New Our Bodies, Ourselves: A Book by and for Women:*

> Much of our ill health as fat women results from the stress of living with fat-hatred—social ridicule and hostility, isolation, financial pressures resulting from job discrimination, lack of exercise due to harassment and, perhaps most important, the hazards of repeated dieting.

There was my life in a nutshell.

"Fat hatred" was a new term to me. It rang true. The realization that sexism, classism and looksism had some power in my life freed me from a burden of guilt I had carried since the age of 11.

Those two little words, "fat hatred," and all the meaning they carried with them, empowered me. Suddenly my life of yo-yo diets, food obsessions, drug abuses and fears of fat made sense.

I'd like to report a full conversion. The truth is that I have had a gradual growth in this area, with spurts and starts. Ten years and a lot of education later, I still have "fat and ugly days" where I'm sure I am the most hideous creature that ever walked the earth and wonder if one last diet wouldn't solve all my problems. But those days are rarer with each passing year.

Even after rejecting the exaggerated claims surrounding the health consequences of being fat and coming to an understanding that health has social and cultural dimensions, I still felt ugly. I was resigned to never being beautiful in the eyes of other people, and thought accepting my ugliness was part of accepting my fat. I understood that fatness might not be the opposite of fitness, but surely it was the opposite of beauty.

I came to regard myself as worthwhile and beautiful *on the inside,* but ugly and misshapen on the outside. I frequently mouthed the words "Fat is Beautiful," but I meant "beautiful on the inside" every time I said them. Beauty was something defined by other people, and no one would ever look at me as beautiful on the outside, I was sure of that.

It turned out, however, that separating health from beauty was a good first step in understanding the social framing of fatness.

Separating health from beauty is difficult to do in our society, especially concerning fatness. Fatness is regarded as neither healthy nor beautiful. Being fat is regarded as a sign of ill health and ugliness. Low body fat, either in the form of the thin figure or the hard-body figure, is regarded as a sign of health and beauty.

Like my student, I regarded beauty as something that radiates *from* the object of admiration. That is how we say it. We say a mountain scene *is* beautiful. We say a woman *is* beautiful.

Then one day, I took a look around and *decided* to see the beauty in other people.

I'm not sure how I got to that moment. I just came to a realization that I could decide for myself what was beautiful and what was not.

Along with women's studies, in my undergrad program I studied visual concepts and had developed my skills as a photographer. I suspect that beginning to see the world as a camera sees it may have had something to do with this realization. But I can't trace a specific line of thought that led me to my moment of discovery of so many beautiful things around me. I just started noticing that things I had never defined as beautiful had qualities I could appreciate.

And as I realized that if I opened my eyes and my heart, I could find beauty in what I observed, I began to accept that others might see beauty in my own fat body.

Beauty does not radiate out of an object. Beauty is truly in the eye of the beholder.

Beauty is something we appreciate in other people, places and things. Beauty is the sum of our beliefs about the value and pleasures those other people, places and things have to offer.

Beauty can be re-evaluated, updated, rethought and renewed.

I am not saying, as the song says, that "everything is beautiful in its own way." I see ugliness in the world. Not *everything* is beautiful. However, seeing beauty where others do not can make a powerful statement about the ugliness of oppression, greed and fear that often cloud human relationships.

My initial love for women's studies has been tempered over the years, because despite some lip service to fat women, many feminists do not question health or beauty statements about fatness. As an active member of a local chapter of the National Organization for Women (NOW), I suffered many conversations about the latest diets and weight loss attempts of members and was approached by several "well-meaning" feminists about my weight. Body image was a problem, to be sure, but it was defined in terms of extreme weight loss attempts. "Sensible" weight loss was an acceptable goal among my feminist friends. The underlying fat hatred inherent in that goal was left unexamined.

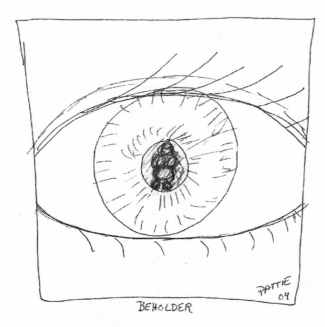

BEHOLDER

Like Orbach's contention 20 years before, I found feminists mostly saw fatness in terms of patriarchal control of women's bodies, with the final goal being a release from patriarchy that would lead to thinness for all women. In a convoluted way, my fatness was regarded as an indication that I had not yet broken the bonds of patriarchy on my life.

This is a view shared by many psychotherapists and mental health counselors. I have sought out psychological counseling on a number of occasions. A few have helped me sort through important personal issues such as coping with rape and with the loss of a child. One was quite good at providing me with knowledge of my cultural context and convincing me not to blame myself for the power limitations placed upon my life as working class and female.

None of them helped me understand fatness as a cultural struggle. Like feminists, every mental health professional I encountered believed that my body weight was indicative of deep emotional issues.

I know there are mental health professionals who are fat-accepting and do not automatically assume fat people have emotional difficulties, or that any emotional difficulties a fat person has are connected to their fatness, or that healing emotional difficulties will lead to weight loss. I have not, however, had the privilege of being a client of a fat-accepting mental health professional.

Making fat a mental illness has many of the same roots as making fat a physical illness. Like physicians, mental health professionals approach stigma from the perspective of a medical model, concentrating most often on what an individual can do to help themselves rather than on the limitations of life chances that the stigma creates. Like physicians, mental health professionals expand their control and their market by expanding definitions of mental illnesses, so making fat psychologically grounded is profitable both in the power sense and in the monetary sense. Like physicians, mental health professionals live within the fishbowl called culture, and may often not question cultural ideas or norms.

On one occasion, I had a chance to read an assessment made of me by a clinical psychologist. I was amazed at the extent to which the language of this report was about how I looked rather than about what I said. To justify her assessment of me as in need of counseling (and, thus, to justify insurance coverage for that counseling), she included statements about how my wearing a sweatshirt and stretch pants indicated "low self-esteem" and that my "frumpy" appearance and being "overweight" indicated "clinical depression." She even discussed how my not wearing makeup indicated the possibility of my being rebellious or socially isolated.

The fact that I had just been laid off from my job, was living on unemployment and food stamps, and wanted to save my good clothes and makeup for job interviews did not appear in her report. She was fully aware of my current economic circumstances, and she could have easily explored how I looked directly with me, but the topic was not raised during her intake interview. I was certainly willing and able to explain my clothing if she had asked.

Even if I were depressed, would it really seem so unreasonable that someone who had just lost her job and was having difficulty finding a new job would be depressed?

I cannot help but believe a thin client would have been assessed much differently. A fat person in a sweatsuit with no makeup is lazy and has no style. A thin person in a sweatsuit and no makeup is comfortable.

From the point I walked into that interview, the counselor was looking for reasons to describe me as mentally ill. My fatness guaranteed that, and if something I said wouldn't do the trick, then something I was wearing might.

It was the feminist counselor who gave me access to this assessment in my record. I asked her if this was a particularly odd narrative for an intake assessment. She indicated to me that indeed appearance is one of the ways that psychologists justify diagnoses and treatments.

Fatness is a symptom used frequently to justify treatment. If this symptom is important even in the absence of other indications of mental illness, it is no wonder there is such a high "correlation" between fatness and mental illness.

It has also been disappointing to find fat politics has just as poor a home on the left as it has on the right. In fact, libertarians and conservatives who reject government involvement with anything deemed personal are often more quickly in bed with fat activists than are leftists who use fatness as a symbol of rampant consumerism and other perceived ills.

Fat people, for many liberals, represent the quintessential American with an insatiable appetite. Fatness and food and laziness and unbridled appetites are bound together symbolically. I am a symbol of over-consumption to these people because of how I look, not because of what I do.

Most fat activists attempt to separate these symbols by challenging medical beliefs. One can be fat and fit. One can be fat and eat health-fully. Fat people are not all lazy. Fat people can be healthy. Fat can even provide protection from some diseases. Dieting can hurt health. Fat people need better medical care. Fat people need places to exercise without being harassed. Fat people need to feel good in and about their bodies.

Only a few activists, however, have challenged the beauty myth head on. Narrow standards of beauty and the place of advertising and media in perpetuating these narrow standards are questioned. The prevalence of eating disorders among young people is often cited. Dating services and special events where fat people can meet each other certainly rely upon a rejection of only certain people as beautiful. The reclamation of the word "fat" is a good step towards questioning narrow standards, but developing a more inclusive aesthetic is rarely on the agenda of most activists.

The culture of consumption that wealthier countries have developed is a culture based on advertising. Advertising is a manipulation of desire and, inevitably, a manipulation of the definitions of beauty. The sad part of using fat people as a symbol of this consumption is that those who would challenge over-consumption have cut themselves off from formidable allies.

The high esteem of thinness is a common means of encouraging over-consumption. In fact, it is an advertiser's wet dream, because dieting does not work most of the time, but it seems to work enough of the time that it encourages consumers to try harder, consume more potions and plans. Thus, it is a product that never satisfies while promising health and beauty, and, therefore, assumedly, happiness and well-being.

Over-consumption has set up a system of producing culture as if the bottom line is all that matters. It is as if the only important cultural icons are those that are produced in conjunction with consumption—that is, promoting mass media and advertising products.

Witness the trend to list films on the basis of their box office receipts rather than quality. Witness the ways in which singers expand their careers via ad campaigns. Witness how product shots in television and film no longer distinguish themselves as ads, but are so integrated into the story lines that few people realize they have been subtly reminded to consume.

Medicine has not escaped this. Celebrities regularly do interviews or talk shows, telling their "personal" stories with health problems, including such things as acid reflux, depression, and weight loss surgery, neglecting to mention that a pharmaceutical company is paying them a "per appearance" fee that can reach five figures.

There is little distinction between our culture and our economy.

1994. Hanging out with Tigger at MGM Studios in Orlando, Florida. This was just the beginning of my journey to self-acceptance. Not waiting to go places until I lost weight was a big step.

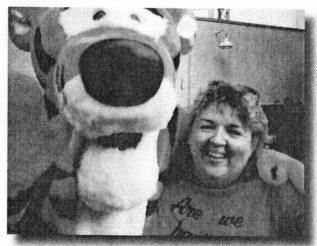

Photo 1994 Carl Wilkerson

They have essentially become equivalent. Economic transactions have become the basis for the shared values we call "culture."

Fighting over-consumption and the co-option of culture by economic concerns should begin with re-evaluating what we believe is desirable. But something more radical is needed to change cultural stereotypes about fat people. What is needed is a radical appreciation for the beauty of people no matter their shape. What is needed is a radical space for the acceptance of people as people as they are *now*, as opposed to *then* or *when*.

This is not some New Age, Pollyanna-ish call for the inner beauty of all spirits, or a romantic pipe dream of a utopian society that might evolve some day. Instead, I am asserting that this radical appreciation needs only a change of mind, a simple decision to really look at people as they are, without the image of some simulated "ideal body" for comparison.

Thus, Step One of the Five Easy Steps to a Beautiful You is to appreciate the beauty of fatness.

Fatness is a reminder that nature loves variety. Fatness is a reminder of the possibility of a bountiful life, a life of plenty rather than a life of constant consumption to make up for what is believed to be lacking. Fatness is a reminder of the joy of being in space and time, taking up a part of the world rather than containing oneself in a pre-designated

115

space. Fatness is a reminder that in spite of efforts by numerous economic interests in the diet-pharmaceutical industrial complex, people can decide for themselves to assess what they enjoy, what they regard as worthwhile.

To appreciate the beauty of fat is to say that I get to decide what I value, what I enjoy, what I want. It is to find my own voice.

I invite you to take the first step and decide for yourself what is beautiful.

Step #2: Resist the negative.

Advertising's influence on media content is exerted in two major ways: via the suppression of information that would harm or "offend the sponsor" and via the inclusion of editorial content that is advertiser-friendly, that creates an environment in which the ads look good. The line between advertising and editorial content is blurred by "advertorials" (advertising disguised as editorial copy), "product placement" in television programs and feature films, and the widespread use of "video news releases," corporate public-relations pull pieces aired by local television stations as genuine news. Up to 85 percent of the news we get is bought and paid for by corporations eager to gain positive publicity.

Jean Kilbourne
media critic & author of *Can't Buy My Love*

I have invented a game that I play when I am particularly bored or in a particularly masochistic mood. The game is called *Flip*.

The rules are simple. A remote control and a television with multiple stations are required to play the game. I start at the beginning of the television channels (usually number two), and I start watching. If some form of fat hatred appears on the screen, I flip to the next channel. I watch for a maximum of five minutes before I move on. So either I flip because I've seen a fat joke, a diet ad, some news story proposing that fat is always bad, or some other anti-fat message, or I flip because the five minutes have passed.

I rarely have to wait the five minutes. The median is probably one minute. I usually can't watch a station for more than a minute without seeing some anti-fat message. This is true on government channels, educational channels, news channels, and so forth. It doesn't seem to matter what the expressed mission of the station is; some anti-fat message will almost always appear before five minutes are up. My record of going through all 58 channels to which I subscribed on cable was about 28 minutes. I don't think I've played a game that lasted over an hour and a half yet.

Take the *Flip* challenge. Go ahead. I dare you. Remember, though, you have to be savvy about what constitutes an anti-fat message. They range from blatant to subtle.

Most frequently I see a diet or fitness commercial or infomercial. Second place goes to fat jokes. They are in style right now, and I rarely tune into a stand-up comedy show or sitcom on which a fat joke doesn't show up fairly quickly. Third place goes to the news story or talk show featuring the "obesity expert" or the "celebrity spokesperson." Next is the comedic and/or dramatic situation in which a fat person is ridiculed, shunned or stereotyped.

I could count the images that promote super-thin bodies, I suppose, but I don't. I could count the images that suggest only the thin are having fun, having sex, getting a good education, obtaining the best jobs, and so forth, but I don't. I could count the commercials that use thin and/or hard bodies to sell everything from toothpaste to financial

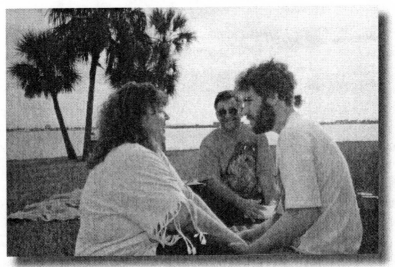

Photo 1992 Peggy Griffin

On October 10, 1992, at sunset, Carl and I said our vows in front of friends and family. This was one of the happiest days of my life.

118

planning, implying that even the money of fat people is no good, but I don't.

The belief that fat is bad and thin is good is marbled so thoroughly into what we see and hear that most of us don't even notice. While the average American is supposedly gaining weight and growing older, the average television show is full of young, thin people.

As media critic Jean Kilbourne aptly points out, the media is selling the audience to advertisers, and the advertisers want 18- to 35-year-olds who have a lot of money, who want to spend that money on images of who they "should" be, and who don't have enough life experience yet to realize that most of that crap won't be very satisfying in the end. Thus, shows that look like that image and sell that image support the products that promote that image.

The image is young, thin, white, straight, with bright teeth and enough wealth to purchase all the products needed to keep the illusion going. There are some variations, but even African-Americans and gay people are often depicted in ways that reflect white and straight values.

As I am writing this, the most talked about show in America is *Friends,* because it is going off the air after 10 years. I'm now happily married to a wonderful man who strives very hard to fight overconsumption in his daily life. He prides himself on never having watched a single episode of *Friends.*

Carl is fond of saying that an easy answer to the mass media problem is to turn off the television. Of course, in an age in which televisions are airing in public places all the time, that is harder than it seems. So when Carl realized about nine years ago that he had successfully remained ignorant of a show that apparently a large number of people were watching, he decided that he would consciously avoid ever seeing the show or learning anything about it. He even flips the channel when he recognizes one of the actors from *Friends* is on another show talking about the show, although his lack of knowledge about *Friends* is so complete that I often have to mention he's watching a *Friends* actor so he can tune them out.

So, 10 years ago he made a decision to remain as ignorant as humanly possible (without going to a cave somewhere) of the whats and wherefores of the show. And in spite of this conscious and deliberate effort, he still knows Jennifer Aniston is on the show. He knows it has three women among the principals. He knows it is set in New York City. He knows the theme song for the show is *I'll Be There for You.*

This is the problem of popular culture: No matter how much you try to tune it out, some of it seeps into your brain. Often you have no memory of where you learned what you know. You just *know.*

Though not as radically opposed to the show as my husband, I quit watching *Friends* a long time ago. I found *Friends* to be one of the most fat-hateful shows on television. This is true not only because one would believe no fat people have ever graced New York if one watched the show, but because the characters consistently degrade fatness, their own fat histories, and fat people. The most infamous example, of course, is the "fat Monica" episodes, where Courtney Cox dons a fat suit to portray her character's high school days and the fat she "outgrew."

I have grown to dislike the fat suit tremendously. I have yet to see or hear of the use of a fat suit that wasn't connected to some form of fat hatred, even with the best of intentions.

I am not alone in my disdain for fat suits. According to Melissa Metzler in her 2001 *Bitch* editorial, fat suits are the new blackface of film:

> A brief history of the fat suit would have to include Goldie Hawn, living large and vengeful in *Death Becomes Her;* Robin Williams—annoying as ever—as chubby, dowdy *Mrs. Doubtfire;* Martin Lawrence and a pair of really weird saggy boobs in *Big Momma's House;* Mike Myers as Fat Bastard in *Austin Powers: The Spy Who Shagged Me;* and Eddie Murphy playing an entire fat family in both *Nutty Professor* movies. More recently, there's Martin Short unable to cross his legs in his new Comedy Central talk show *Primetime Glick,* Julia Roberts scarfing down cookies as a (gasp!) size 12 in *America's Sweethearts,* and a fat-family dream sequence on Damon Wayan's sitcom *My Wife and Kids.* Fat people are now America's favorite celluloid punchlines. Wanna make a funny movie? It's a pretty easy formula: Zip a skinny actor

into a latex suit. Watch her/him eat, walk, and try to find love. Hilarity will ensue. [1]

At the risk of sounding "too serious," I find this kind of comedy disturbing because it reinforces so many of the horrible things people think about bodies like mine and the character of the people who occupy those bodies. It reinforces the whole notion that my fatness is something I *wear* rather than a part of my body. It suggests that under every fat person is a thin person waiting to emerge. My experience as a fat person is never reflected in these fat impersonations.

There have been others who have worn fat suits in recent years. Anita Roddick, the CEO and founder of The Body Shop, decided in 2002 to put on a fat suit to see how it felt to be fat. On her web site, she reports:

> As a very active person who finds it impossible to sit still, I found the weight restricting and uncomfortable. I hated not being able to move quickly. My life has never been sedentary. I've always found huge breasts slightly disconcerting, the way they get in the way of running and moving. Being short at 5 ft 2 in, I'm even less able to carry weight. I just seem to expand outwards. The heaviest I've ever been was when carrying my daughters in pregnancy. During the filming I could only wear the suit for a few hours a day because I found it so frustrating and physically grueling.

Certainly her motives were different from the actors listed earlier. Roddick seems sincere in her desire to understand the experience of being fat. She drew several conclusions from her experiences that seem sensitive enough. But like the actors, Roddick confuses the experience of a fat *suit* with the experience of being fat. A fat suit no more simulates the experience of fatness than painting one's face with black shoe polish makes one an expert on being African American.

What surprised me most about Roddick's experiment is how body-centered it was. If she truly wanted to understand the experience of being treated like a second-class citizen because of her size, then her comments, interviews and film would have been about the social interaction she encountered, not about the fat suit and the physical limitations of being fat.

In other words, the experiment could have been a good social experiment, but it was, and remained, a lousy biological one. Roddick concentrated on her physical experience. She reported her difficulties with heat, mobility, and using the washroom more than she did about the social treatment she received as a larger person. Rather than going to public places where fat people would be shunned, she opted for fat-friendly venues. Her interests were in understanding the oppressed, not the oppressor, an arrangement always fraught with difficulties.

Even with the best intentions, the wearing of a fat suit reinforces a extremely pervasive and negative idea about fat bodies—the idea that fat is something that resides on the outside of the "real" body. This is a widely held belief. The thinner "you" residing inside a layer of fat is supposedly the truer self, that part of you that wants to emerge if only whatever problems that keep you fat would (and this is the word usually used in this context) "melt" away.

It is a powerful story. I have told this story during my personal weight loss experiences.

Somewhere in the world, I am a success story in a collection of success stories for a bariatric clinic. I lost 130 pounds using the clinic's methods. I wish I had access to exactly what I wrote in my "success story" letter. It has been lost over the years, and I have no desire to contact the clinic, if it indeed still exists, and ask them for the letter. I remember, however, writing something to the effect that as the pounds melted off my body and I found my thin inner self, I was only able to be successful because along with the outer fat I shed my pain, fear and shame.

I believe the letter left out the part about getting addicted to speed and Valium. I know it left out that within five years I gained back the 130 pounds, plus another 40 or so pounds. Even if I took the time to write a follow-up letter, I'm certain *that* testimonial would never make into their ads.

Mass media weight loss accounts are full of omissions such as the weight being gained back and then some. Most reporters will never question the long-term effects of "successful" dieting programs. Most editors will never assign a reporter to follow-up weight loss stories.

Oh, sure, a few stories about the horrors of drastic dieting will show up when a celebrity such as Mary-Kate Olsen checks into an eating disorder clinic. Speculations on which of the thinnest of the stars is bulimic or anorexic are a major preoccupation with celebrity media. A few anti-weight-loss surgery stories are appearing now that a few people have suffered complications and death, but these are unsurprising considering the economic interests of insurance companies that do not like paying for highly risky surgeries that can't be shown to improve lifestyles or their bottom-lines.

Most of the true stories of dieting are never published in the media because the diet industry is a billion-dollar industry that advertises in every form of media that exists. That means most forms of media will want to present an audience that is interested in dieting to this billion-dollar customer That, in turn, means the media will present characters, plot lines and images that attract and encourage an audience to make weight loss a goal.

In the mass media, the audience is the product being sold to advertisers, and where diet ads are concerned, the product is an audience dissatisfied and confused about their own bodies. That is what the phenomenal success of *Friends* is about, selling an audience the ideal that these six young people represent.

Monica's fat history is the party line on fatness. Inside every fat teenager is a Monica ready to bloom. Melt away the fat suit and you can be Monica, too—not entirely satisfied with yourself, but certainly successful enough to buy the things you need to make yourself presentable to a judging world.

After all, it is not *satisfaction* you are being taught. The media wants to sell a *dissatisfied* audience to those producers of goods that may satisfy enough to make you feel better, but never satisfy quite so much that you will not keep buying more.

How can anyone feel beautiful in this kind of atmosphere? Are we all doomed to a lifeless world without celebration or makeup in order to fight the overwhelming desire to consume the latest whatever-makes-you-feel-good?

On the surface, that seems to be the choice. On the one hand, we can consume, knowing full well we are being manipulated through a media that wants us to be a dissatisfied audience so it can sell us to their advertisers. On the other hand, we can become the ascetic, never watching, listening to or reading media, dropping out of pop culture altogether.

How can we resist the negative?

I suggest that we do not have to follow the path of the ignorant over-consumer automaton who buys all it is told to buy. Nor do we have to follow the path of the ascetic who refuses to have any fun for fear of falling prey to the sins of over-consumption.

I offer three other options to resist the negative:

1. *Become media literate.* Understand how the media work, why they work, and for whom they work. Specifically, understand that you, the audience, are the product about which the media are most concerned. If a certain show appeals to you, question what audience the media are selling to the advertisers. Ask yourself why you like a particular show and if you are being manipulated into watching through slick production values, attractive stars and so forth. Pay attention to who is advertising during this time.

   Knowing the game helps to resist the game. The game works, in part, because advertising and story lines are enchanting. Nothing disenchants faster than seeing underneath the façade.

2. *Turn off media that offend you.* I am always amazed at the number of people who continue to watch or read or listen to media they find offensive. The endless discussions in popular press regarding censorship are a smoke and mirrors game that convinces people they cannot simply choose what they watch in their own homes. We do not need regulations. We need people who know how to turn a switch, pull a plug, or hit a delete key. Continuing to watch or listen to media that offends you makes you one of

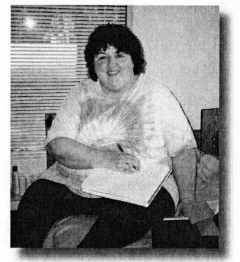

1999.
Wild Women's
Weekend Retreat.

This was my preparation
for my qualifying exams—
I decided I needed to renew my
spirit and strengthen my mind.

those morbid rubber-neckers who hold up traffic to check out the carnage.

Your brain is a learning machine. It is constantly picking up information through your five senses—touch, taste, smell, hearing, and sight. Media production is designed to stimulate those senses and provide your brain with information. If you don't like the information you are being offered, cut off the source. Most media run on electricity, and electricity is easy to put under your control. The only knowledge you need to have is where the plug or switch is. There are so many media you can't escape, take advantage of the opportunities in which you *can* escape.

3. ***Pay attention to your own life experiences and honor them.*** Most people are susceptible to the media messages they receive because they are starved for attention, love and understanding. Resisting the negative can be difficult if the negative is embodied in a message that promises attention, love and understanding.

If you can find more positive ways to give yourself attention, love and understanding, you won't be vulnerable to these ads. In other words, you will be more satisfied with your life, and satisfaction is the remedy for sales vulnerability. The more satisfied you are under your own skin, the less likely it will be that some product will appeal to you.

Salesmen begin with teaching you to be dissatisfied. They have to convince you of a need before they can convince you they have the answer for your need. Living a fulfilling life often means going against all the advice you have been given, because most of the advice you have been given is meant to keep you dissatisfied so you will purchase more.

Question everything. The more you know yourself and your own sense of satisfaction, the less you will want to buy. You won't be gullible anymore.

I know that these three things are more difficult than they seem. I struggle with the negotiation between consumption and asceticism daily, even years after becoming aware of the purpose and processes of media production. But resisting the negative is an important second step towards a beautiful you. It is the way you make your decision stick.

If you get to decide what is beautiful, then you must resist having beauty defined for you by others.

Step #3: Talk the talk.

We have elevated the pursuit of a lean, fat-free body into a new religion. It has a creed: I eat right, watch my weight, and exercise."
Indeed the anorexia nervosa could be called the paradigm of our age, for our creed encourages us all to adopt the behavior and attitudes of the anorexic. The difference is one of degree, not of kind. Like any religion worthy of the name, ours also has its damnation. Failure to follow the creed—and the corporeal stigmata of that failure, fatness and flabbiness—produce a hell on earth. The fat and flabby are damned to failure, regardless of professional and personal successes. Our religion also has it rewards, its salvation. In following the creed, one is guaranteed beauty, energy, health, and a long, successful life. Followers are even promised self-transformation: The "thin person within," waiting to burst through the fat, is somehow a more exciting, sexy, competent, successful self.

Roberta P. Seid
historian & author of *Never Too Thin*

When most people think about disease, they think about bugs. Little itty-bitty germs that wreak havoc on human beings along a continuum that begins with mild annoyances up to deadly bleeding-from-the-eyes horrors. It seems like a very simple proposition. What is good for some of those microscopic organisms *ain't* good for us humans. So a disease is an easy concept, right? A bug *invades* and a doctor prescribes something that a person ingests or absorbs that will *fight* the infection. If the medication is good, the bug dies and the person gets well.

Diseases, however, are far more complex than the bug scenario would lead us to believe. Diseases like autoimmune disorders defy the germ theory of disease because the body seems to turn on itself, attacking good cells as if they were bugs, often with no visible foreign invader present.

Genetics also complicate the picture, because one germ can be devastating to one person's health with little or no effect on another person. How strong a person's immune system is will also determine the efficacy of medications. Not all medicines work in the same way for all people.

Not only is the physiology more complex, but medicine and medical research are done by human beings, and human beings live within a fishbowl we call "culture." There is no escaping that culture, even with the noblest of scientific callings and the best of scientific procedure. The second a physical phenomenon is named, it gains a cultural context. Discoveries and findings of scientific research must be reported to others in order to be of value. Reporting means using language. Language always has a cultural context. It is unavoidable.

Choice of research topic also limits scientific research as a whole. By choosing to study one thing, a scientist effectively rejects numerous other things that could be studied. Having a variety of scientists with a variety of interests helps offset this problem, but as long as the interests of funding sources take precedence, certainly many phenomena will remain unstudied. A rare set of symptoms that do not affect a large number of people is often ignored because no scientist is aware of its existence, or because no scientist will gain tenure studying something that has so little impact on the public at large, or because no funding source has figured out a way to make money off it.

In addition, the research question that is formulated precludes other possible questions within the same topic, which is often a deliberate measure on the part of funding sources that have market agendas as well as scientific ones.

For the past 25 years, conventional approaches to treating a condition called "clinical depression" have been influenced by a 50-year-old theory that brain chemistry imbalances are the central cause of the symptoms. The original studies looking at these connections were not conclusive, but pharmaceutical companies latched onto the theory in the 1980s as the basis for their development of powerful antidepressants now prescribed to millions of North Americans. Nowadays, most studies conducted on depression assume the brain chemistry theory and test only for the efficacy of antidepressants in reducing or changing brain chemicals, rather than asking any questions directly about the effect on the patient's moods. It is assumed that if the brain chemistry changes, the patient's mood will also change, but there is a growing body of evidence that the relationship should not be taken for granted.[2]

The choice of research topic and question are only the first in a series of choices that affect the outcome and influence of scientific research. The design of a study and the length of time over which a study is conducted are highly influenced by funding. Well-funded studies are generally longer, larger in scope, and involve more test subjects. While some grants are set up to encourage purer forms of research, most funding comes with agendas. This puts pressure on the researcher to achieve certain outcomes in line with their funding agencies' agendas. Often, further research monies are tied to pleasing the funding source.

As a researcher who worked on publicly funded projects, my experience in writing research reports was that there was a fine political line drawn on what could and could not be reported and/or the style in which the report was written. We did not write patently false reports, but there were ways of saying things that were sensitive to the agendas involved up the line of bureaucracy. Failures to write sufficiently sensitive treatises were met with rejection and calls for rewrites of the reports or threats of withdrawal of funding for future work. It only took me a couple of rewrites to figure out what was acceptable and what wasn't, and my future reports were reflective of those lessons.

After a while, no one had to correct me; I edited myself knowing full well that some salient points were being lost. These points were sometimes discussed orally at conferences or meetings, but they never found their way into written form. Thus, people outside the loop would be hard-pressed to know some of the findings or the implications of those findings. I expect my experience was typical in this respect.

For most scientific research, the reporting of results happens through scientific journals and a process called "peer review." There is some merit to a peer review system. It ensures that qualified people who are familiar with a particular subject can read and understand a particular report. It ensures that what is published in a journal has a certain air of legitimacy because it has been scrutinized before release.

While most journals do not tell the peer reviewer the name of the researcher(s) who wrote the report, some filtering occurs before the review. Most journals are leery of publishing reports from unaffiliated sources, meaning from people who are not connected with an academic, government or research facility. Such papers are usually rejected without being distributed for peer review at all. Also, papers not printed in the standard formats of the journal, papers not meeting the required page length, and papers deemed not in keeping with the specialization of the journal will be sent back to the author without review.

Buckminster Fuller, most popularly known as the inventor of the geodesic dome, was a highly innovative and respected engineer who dropped out of school and was never affiliated with a university. This made it impossible for him to publish his projects in respected scientific journals. Even though Fuller patented hundreds of inventions, he never sought remedy when his inventions were copied or adopted by other people. His philosophy was that each of his inventions was for the good of humanity, not his own personal profit.

Why did he patent, then? Fuller discovered the opportunity that the patenting application process gave him to document his thinking and discoveries. His patent applications left nothing out, and were full disclosures of his process, outcomes and conclusions. He had to do this because the "purer" scientific forums kept him out not on the basis of how good the science he created was, but on the basis of his credentials.

Even though he is now regarded as one of the most forward thinking inventors of the 20th century, Fuller was simply not part of the social club called "scientists." One is left wondering how many other bits of scientific information are absent from the literature because the source of the discovery or process happened to be outside that social group.

After the initial filtering, the peers asked to review submitted work are usually chosen because of familiarity with similar works that have been published. If a literature review in a report includes a prominent scholar in the field, that scholar is often asked to review the report. This means that studies whose results conflict or negate a scholar's work may be reviewed more negatively in order to protect her or his own body of work. While this practice is frowned upon explicitly, most human beings cannot help but be more critical when their results are questioned or refuted, and less critical when their results are confirmed. Reputation is an important aspect of reward within the tenure system of most universities, even after achieving tenure. Even in government and independent research facilities, reputation means more funding, higher salaries, more research assistants, and more publications. It is hard to imagine that researchers would not be susceptible to these social and organizational concerns.

Many studies are not published because the researchers never submit their work for publication. Results that conflict with well-known studies, results that are different from the anticipated outcome, or results that are mixed and present no clear picture are often rejected by the researcher, who "goes back to the drawing board" rather than let people know about the less conclusive research. This means that those studies that get published reflect on a select few of all the research being conducted in a given scientific area.

Finally, it should be noted that even published reports are subject to skepticism and scrutiny. Research reports usually have five sections to them: introduction, literature review, data, results, and discussion.

2000.
Carl and I in
Minneapolis, in a
friend's garden on
the trip west
to Victoria,
British Columbia,
where I visited
at the Centre on
Aging and wrote
my dissertation.

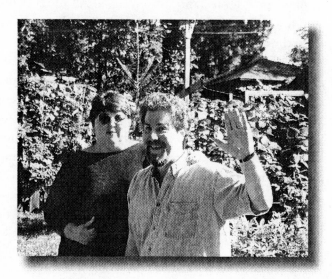

Often peers reviewing the report depend upon the logic of the results and discussion section rather than re-testing or heavily scrutinizing the data section. Results outlined can discuss certain findings while minimizing other findings. Discussions are basically interpretive in nature. All too often, the press release, abstract, or quick perusal of a report depends heavily upon the discussion and offers little chance to review the data fully.

The purer faith of science demands a thorough scrutinizing of data, but most researchers who quote other research do not take the time to do a thorough scrutiny. Thus, even reports on published studies are often misleading or misunderstood.

I am not making a case for letting go of scientific research. I personally believe that medical science has prolonged my life many times over.

I had six years of positive Pap smears with no symptoms whatsoever of the potential cancer cells growing in my cervix. The invention of the Pap smear has saved millions of women from cervical cancer and early death. The pathological testing of skin moles also saved my life because I had a melanoma (the most deadly kind of skin cancer) removed before it spread or became dangerous to me.

I take medications daily that help me maintain my health in spite of asthma, lupus, and fibromyalgia. All of these medications were developed in the atmosphere I described above. I am a walking, talking testimonial to the good work done in medicine.

However, that does not mean science and medicine are conducted without procedural flaws. Nor does my criticism of such systems mean the rejection of these systems as a whole. On the contrary, I agree with social critic and author Sandra Harding[3] when I assert that understanding the cultural contexts to the way medical knowledge comes into being makes me a more informed consumer of medicine, and makes scientific research more complete.

Traditionally, scientific method has been seen as something "objective" and "neutral." While no one argues that achieving these goals is 100 percent possible, these are cherished objectives and are thought to be the aim of all scientific endeavors. Harding argues that the consideration of the cultural contexts to the generation of scientific knowledge lends a more solid basis for that knowledge rather than undermining it.

Harding suggests that neutrality is not the same thing as objectivity. Objectivity comes from examining and admitting to the cultural, social, and emotional contexts in which science is developed. Using a concept called *strong objectivity,* she argues that knowing these contexts in the process of a particular study will lead to a better understanding of that study and its topic.

All scientific projects, she argues, are enhanced by reflecting upon the social and cultural forces that created the project. After all, science should not be a religion where doubt is a sign of lost faith. Doubt is central to faith in medicine, because without doubt one could not further knowledge. Harding writes:

> Yet science always promised something better than truth. It has always been understood that what makes a claim a scientific one, and not a matter of political dogma or religious faith, is that it is in perpetuity held open to revision on the basis of future, possibly disconfirming, observations and/ or revisions in the conceptual frameworks of the sciences. The abandonment in scientific circles of the concept of the crucial experiment in the late nineteenth century reflected the recognition that no empirical observations could prove a hypothesis true; (at most) they could only show it to be less false than its known competitors.[4]

What many people do not realize is that diseases or disorders come in and out of style as cultural attitudes change.

Diseases and disorders have been used to justify sexism by asserting that women could not benefit from a college education because they bled once a month, draining the blood from the brain that was needed for thinking.

Diseases and disorders have been used to justify racism by asserting that skull shape, jaw shape, size of lips and eyes and so forth are indicative of mental disorders that lead to lives of crime or indicate a lack of intelligence.

Diseases and disorders have been used to justify classism by suggesting that high libidos and lower intelligence lead to poverty, justifying a "treatment" that has included the forced sterilization of millions of poor and uneducated women.

Barry Glassner, sociologist and author of *Culture of Fear*, points out that in the history of medicine there have been many diseases or disorders that reflect cultural and social conflicts and upheavals rather than the discovery of a particular biological process. He calls these "metaphorical illnesses."

He is not suggesting that the symptoms experienced by the patients are not real, but rather that the interpretations of the physical phenomena are grounded more solidly in the anxieties, misgivings and prejudices of the contemporary society than in the biology of the symptoms. He cites neurasthenia as an example:

> Diagnosed in the United States mostly during the nineteenth century and disproportionately in women, the symptoms of neurasthenia were said to include extreme fatigue, muscle aches, mental confusion, chills, and fever...neurasthenics were not, by and large, hypochondriacs. They were verifiably sick, sometimes seriously so... Back in 1881, however, George Beard, the physician known as the "father of neurasthenia," attributed the illness to modern technology and the education of women. Then as now, people believed in metaphoric illnesses partly owing to graphic stories about ordinary women and men being struck down and partly because the illnesses helped them justify fears, prejudices, and political ideologies they held. The disease of neurasthenia provided living, breathing proof that newly developed technologies and women's emancipation truly *were* pernicious."[5]

I believe obesity is a metaphorical illness that will someday be debunked. This belief, I know, is tantamount to heresy in the current religious fervor that is the war on fat. This belief, I know, is especially easy to ignore coming from a fat woman. Nonetheless, the creation of this disease, the controversies surrounding the medical studies and the public discussions of this disease are not unlike those characteristic of predecessors such as neurasthenia.

There is no doubt that the average Westerner has more body mass than his counterparts in earlier generations. Certainly, a correlation exists between larger body mass and certain health conditions. But a risk factor is a far cry from a cause.

Many others have attacked the "obesity" issue from a medical point of view, and I will not repeat their arguments here.[6] My concern here is a question of beauty, not health.

Three specific social situations are at work in the creation of obesity as a disease: (1) patient pressure, (2) the process of patenting medicine, and (3) the long history of marketing "cures" for fatness. While these three social situations have medical language and medical overtones to their interactions, at the base of each of these interactions is a question of fashion, not medicine.

Many times a disease is named because doctors feel *patient pressure* to give a set of symptoms a label. Patients and their family members who suffer from life-interrupting and life-threatening symptoms often seek out the legitimacy of medical designations for their particular circumstances because they are more likely to receive medical attention and health care coverage when such designations exist. For this reason, many diseases or disorders emerge from patient demand for a name for their symptoms.

Personally, I understand this need for naming ailments.

In March 1997 I became violently ill, throwing up to the point of dehydration. I thought at the time that I had caught a bug or had food poisoning. The violent symptoms passed, but I did not get better. I lacked energy, yet I couldn't sleep at all. My joints ached constantly, and I was taking so much aspirin to relieve the pain that my ears were constantly ringing.

Test after test was conducted to assess my condition, but the results all were negative. I was at my wits' end by August, when I finally received a diagnosis: lupus. Upon being told that I had an incurable disease that I would have to live with for the rest of my life and could possibly shorten my life, I felt relief. Finally, I had a name for what was wrong, and with that name came a way of coping with the symptoms.

When the symptoms were nameless, I felt lost and ostracized. A name meant that I could receive certain services, I could explain certain behaviors, I could opt out of specific responsibilities, and I could expect a certain future.

This sense of relief, according to Kathy Charmez in her book *Good Days, Bad Days,* is not unusual. A number of the chronically ill people she interviewed for her study reported that after lengthy testing and months, maybe even years, of not knowing, they felt an overwhelming sense of relief once their condition was named.

The pioneering American sociologist Talcott Parsons in the 1950s offered an interesting explanation for this seemingly illogical reaction. He describes the relationship between health care worker and patient in terms of the roles they play in society.

The patient is in what he called the *sick role.* In our society, when one is sick, one is given a way to excuse oneself from other roles, and one is given the chance to get well. Opposite the sick role is the role of the health care worker, usually a physician in our society. The professional health care worker is in the *physician role,* a role expected to be played with aloofness, expertise and effectiveness. Physicians are supposed to know all the things that patients do not know about medical conditions. Both roles have certain responsibilities, certain powers, and certain limitations.

This description of the physician/patient interaction works beautifully under the bug theory of illness. The physician has gone to school and worked as an apprentice for many years, allowing her or him often to recognize symptoms instantly and know the exact cure to offer the patient. The patient's responsibility is to take her or his medicine and follow "doctor's orders" in an effort to get well. The special privileges both are afforded in this social interaction only continue if the doctor can make the patient well and the patient makes every effort to get well.

A diagnosis or named disease sets up a social interaction that is easy to follow and rewards both the sick and the physician. It is one of the more powerful relationships in our society. A physician can make it possible for a designated sick person to be excused from work or school with pay and without penalty. A physician can make it possible for a designated sick person to receive disability benefits, government aid, and other kinds of funding. A physician can make it possible for a designated sick person to hold special privileges such as parking at the front of a lot or not having to do housework.

Of course, the designated sick person has to be making an effort to get well within a reasonable amount of time. If the doctor cannot name the disease and the patient cannot get well in a finite amount of time, the relationship and its acceptability in society at large becomes more complex. Chronically ill people are often shunned and ostracized and begin to lose their privileges over time. Even terminally ill people and elderly people are shunned and are often expected to keep to themselves and their families until "the end."

However, the *sick role* has traditionally offered protections for people who otherwise would be considered deviant. Sympathy and social services are offered to the sick that are not offered to the "weird," the "criminal," or the "shy." Being sick engenders a certain amount of sympathy. It is not unlimited sympathy, but it is more sympathy than other deviant roles evoke.[7] So, even with the risk of eventually being ostracized, there is a strong incentive for patients to demand diagnoses and treatments from physicians, and there is a strong incentive for physicians to provide such diagnoses and treatments even if there is no medical or scientific evidence to support them.

Peter N. Stearns, in *Fat History*, found that the first records of doctors prescribing diets were a result of fashion, not science. In the 1920s, when flat-chested flapper girls were the beauties of the age, many middle class women went to their physicians demanding methodologies to lose weight. Much of the early medical literature on dieting was concerned with finding healthy ways for women to be "stylishly slender."

Stearns also points out that complicating this demand was the fact that physicians were human beings who were affected by the whims of fashion as well. Doctors began to regard fatness as a sign of weakness and ugliness. This prejudice was reinforced by the fact that most people failed to lose weight or stick to the dietary guidelines being prescribed.

So, basically, the demand for weight loss strategies by middle class women who wanted to be fashionably thin led to a rejection of the sick role for those fat people who simply could not or would not lose weight. In this case, as in the general case, in order to enjoy the privileges of being sick, one had to stick to the treatment and eventually become well. But dieting is notoriously ineffective. Physicians, protecting their professional territories, started distinguishing between patients who had "glandular problems" and patients who were healthy but overweight. The latter group was described, in a burst of circular logic, as having "indolence obesity," because it was assumed that their fatness indicated they were not following doctor's orders.

For a physician to treat patient demand, at some point there had to be a disease or disorder or medical risk to justify the expertise the physician role demanded. Scientific study was needed to justify the advice given in the office.

From the beginning, the questions being asked in the laboratory about fatness were aimed at defining the relationship between fatness and illness. No one has ever studied fatness just to understand fatness. The subject has always been tackled as a "problem" that requires a "cure." This means that a bias has been built into the study of fatness even before the actual experiments began. This bias was dictated by fashion, not scientific discovery.

Once the "fat-is-a-disease" ball got rolling, other social forces moved it along. A particularly strong organizational force was and is the process for patenting medicine.

In the United States and Canada, a drug patent is an extremely valuable asset. Early in the research process, a pharmaceutical company will apply for a patent, which gives the company exclusive rights to use the chemical compound over the next 20 years to develop and distribute the substance, pending approval by the government agencies in charge of drug safety. The patent must state what the substance contains and for what, specifically, the substance will be used.

A good part of that 20 years is spent gaining approval from the appropriate government agency. The onus is on the company to convince the government agency that the drug is effective and relatively safe. Once an average drug hits the market, it will have around seven years left of its monopoly. The end of that monopoly means a substantial lowering of the profitability of sales due to the fact that generic versions, competitive versions, and over-the-counter versions will most likely appear to compete with the sales of the original version.

The monopoly is deemed necessary because the process by which a safe and effective medication hits the market is very long and requires a great deal of expense in research and presentation of results. There are many medications that do not get approval after many years and much money, so it seems fair to allow these companies who take such risks for the public good to be able to recoup losses and accumulate gains in order to further medical research.

On the surface, this seems reasonable, but there are some built-in incentives in the system that lead to distortions of the pretty picture of research and development. Pharmaceutical companies are rewarded when their patents are extended. Two powerful strategies available to them to extend patents have implications for obesity research: reformulation and fast track approval.

When a company applies for a patent, it must state for what the invention, substance or idea will be used. One way to extend a patent is to reformulate the invention, substance or idea. Another is to reformulate the use of the invention, substance or idea. Several medications on the market have used "treatment" of "obesity" as a way to extend the benefits of their patents. Probably the best known are two medications that were approved in the 1990s by the FDA: Redux and Meridia. Though they worked in different ways, both of these medications were reformulations of previous medications that had been around for many years.

Pondimin (fenfluramine) was approved in 1973 as a means to increase body levels of the neurotransmitter serotonin by preventing or slowing the natural breakdown of serotonin, keeping the levels in the body higher. It was recommended for short-term use to elevate mood.

The use of fenfluramine in tangent with the amphetamine phentermine (a combination popularly known as phen-fen) was not approved by the FDA, though each drug had been separately approved as safe.

Redux was a patent of the substance dexfenfluramine, which was essentially a reformulation of the mood-elevator fenfluramine into a weight-loss drug. Redux's approval in the midst of reported problems with phen-fen represents one of the more shameful episodes in FDA history.

Meridia (sibutramine) is also a reformulation of a class of drugs known as "selective serotonin reuptake inhibitors," which include well-known antidepressants such as Prozac, Zoloft and Luvox. Sibutramine was first explored as an antidepressant in the late 1980s, making it a latecomer to the SSRI crowd. Knoll Pharmaceuticals, now a part of Abbott Laboratories, chose to explore the weight loss potential rather than the antidepressant qualities of the substance. By 1997, Meridia was approved as a means to reduce weight.

Like phen-fen, both Redux and Meridia have caused a great deal of damage to the health of patients who have tried to lose weight. The FDA issued a warning regarding the use of Redux in 1997, around the same time it issued a warning regarding the use of phen-fen. A number of states subsequently banned the use of phen-fen and Redux. Meridia is currently banned in much of Europe, but it is still available in the United States, though the recommendations for use are much more restricted than originally outlined. Class action suits regarding these drugs have been filed and litigated since 1997.[8]

Another way pharmaceutical companies ensure more profitability is to speed up the approval process in the name of treating an epidemic or serious public health problem. Government agencies that oversee the approval processes of drugs are often under pressure to be quick about it because lives are at risk. One strategy pharmaceutical companies use is to make the case that even when new medications have serious potential side effects, the risk of dying or being disabled from the disease or disorder being treated is greater than the dangers posed by the medications supposed to treat it. This case is made both in the public hearings that are held for gathering evidence to determine the disposition of the drug and in the media, where public pressure can be generated to push for approval.

Such public pressure has been useful when governments have ignored politically charged medical crises like the AIDS epidemic. Lives have been saved or prolonged because of fast track approvals of innovative medications aimed at improving the lives of AIDS victims. The case for obesity, however, is not as strong as the case for AIDS. Full-blown AIDS carries a death sentence that to date no one has been able to escape. Waiting a year or two extra to approve a potentially effective AIDS drug means thousands of people could die while waiting. Terminally ill people are far more willing to be guinea pigs for experimental medications because they have little to lose in the effort.

It is that kind of desperation that obesity researchers and the pharmaceutical companies that fund them hope to create in the public mind in order to generate pressure for fast track approvals. Redux was one of their commercial successes, at least for about a year, after which time its failings in all other respects were apparent.

Despite the problems being reported with the "cocktail" of phen-fen, which had become popular after a 1992 study showed some weight loss benefits when the drugs were used in tandem, Redux had been put on the fast track for FDA approval. Two objections were raised during the approval hearings involving possible problems with pulmonary hypertension and brain damage, and the FDA's own advisory committee initially voted against approving the drug by a close six to five decision.

The FDA changed its mind about Redux, however, after hearing about research done by JoAnn Manson that led them to believe that 30 people would be spared a premature death due to obesity for every one person who died from primary pulmonary hypertension (PPH) caused by Redux. Manson defended her research conclusions even after it was discovered that the number of PPH deaths in patients who took Redux were three times higher than originally reported.

It turned out that Manson was a consultant for Interneuron Pharmaceuticals, the company that developed Redux. This conflict of interest was not mentioned either at the FDA hearings or in a subsequent editorial published in the *New England Journal of Medicine*.

It would be wrong to assume, however, that the FDA caved simply

141

because of Manson's questionable research. The demand for treatments for obesity comes from the public as well, and many obesity researchers use that demand to their advantage. Laura Fraser, in her book *Losing It,* quotes Michael Fumento in reaction to the FDA panel's decision: "In its caution the FDA panel refused to weigh the slight possibility of harm of the drug versus the very real harm caused by obesity…What the heck is going on here? Is the FDA staffed at the highest levels by men who are into fat women?"[9]

Fumento's words are indicative of the cultural context to the FDA's continued desire to fast track medications and procedures aimed at weight loss. The appeal Fumento made was an appeal to desire and preference, not to medicine.

"Into fat women" is meant to be an indictment, and it is one that I find particularly insulting. These words do not inspire me to believe that Fumento is interested in the health of fat women at all. It is the supposed ugliness of fat, not the unhealthiness of fat, that informs his argument.

The underlying assumption in his statement is that "everybody knows" finding fat women desirable is unusual and deviant. Given that, there is little point to fussing around with scientific testing or the results thereof to the extent that they undermine the claim that such prejudice is based in the rational.

It is hard to believe that the cultural disdain for fatness has nothing to do with the FDA's decision-making process. It certainly has something to do with the public demand for medicines like Redux. The miracle pill is sought for beauty, not health. Even the process by which American health is to be protected is influenced by the equivalence of health with beauty.

In the end, thousands of people died or were permanently damaged because of the use of phen-fen and Redux. The list continues to grow of the people who are dying or hurting because of Meridia. The only justification for these numbers can be equating fatness with a "killer" disease.

The events of the past 15 years make it infeasible for obesity researchers, government regulators, and the dieting public to admit that fatness might *not* be harmful. A strong organizational investment has been made in the story that fat is a disease or, at least, a symptom of a disease. It is not surprising most obesity researchers won't even entertain the idea that the relationship between fatness and disease is weak and possibly spurious.[10]

Defining fatness as a disease called "obesity" and then marketing "cures" for fatness in the form of diets, supplements, medications, procedures, and exercise regimens can be an extremely lucrative proposition. The belief that fat is bad, ugly and unwanted fuels what is widely reported as a 30- to 40-billion-dollar per year industry. Most of these claims are pretty easy to spot (what the FTC calls "facially questionable claims"), but even the more legitimate claims tap into these cultural beliefs about fat.

What all weight-loss products, schemes, services and gadgets have in common is a belief that fat is unwanted. To justify this attack on fat, the industry repeats claims about the relationship between fat and disease, often to the point of asserting that fat *is* a disease. Even within such claims, however, "obesity" remains ill-defined and elusive.

One such example of this rhetoric is the case of MLN4760.

In November 1997, Millennium Pharmaceuticals and Abbott Laboratories announced the development of a new genetically based medication that was said to speed up metabolism. The press release and subsequent news coverage of the announcement merits a look, because the miracle-drug story was picked up by news agencies around the world.

The original announcement reported that the drug was being developed to treat "obesity, diabetes, and other metabolic disorders." The implied meaning of obesity changed several times in the press release, and it was never once given an explicit definition.

At first, the disease in question was a "diet-induced-obesity" and was related to diabetes. The drug was said to be for diabetics, who often gain weight either before or after onset of their disease. However, two paragraphs later, obesity became a "serious health concern" with "97 million people" predisposed to "morbid consequences." The press release described Type 2 diabetes, affecting 15.7 million people, as one of those morbid consequences. Despite this difference of 80 million or so people (and that difference is computationally accurate only if you assume that every diabetic is overweight or obese, which is not true), "diabetes" and "obesity" remained paired throughout the remainder of the press release. Both were said to benefit from research on "gene targets" identified as key to "satiety, fat absorption and energy metabolism." According to the press release, the mechanism of MLN4760 was to increase glucose sensitivity in order to stimulate more production of insulin. But that mechanism has nothing to do with fat absorption and only marginally concerns satiety.

Like a magic trick with sleight of hand, right before the reader's eyes *all* fat people have developed metabolic disorders, *all* fat people have induced their fatness through their diet, and *all* "excess" weight leads to morbid consequences. No documentation was offered to back these implied claims. No taxonomy was offered suggesting that fatness may be experienced differently by different people.

The language was scientific, but the transformation was magical. Obesity was a given, an ill-defined, yet supposedly medically sound, given.

Metabolic diseases were singularly addressed in the press release because Millennium and Abbott are makers of metabolic pharmaceuticals. Economics, not biological discovery, drove the press release. It was picked up by *The Wall Street Journal* and addressed to stockholders and potential investors.

The press release was intended to help secure a financial future with a product they hope to sell to a market. A market with 97 million potential customers was preferable to one with 15.7 million. Thus, rhetorically making this drug into something that *all* "overweight" and "obese" people would use was in the best interest of the company. Key to selling this cure was the transformation of body fat into a metabolic disorder.

The Wall Street Journal (November 28, 2001) article included not only the information from the press release, but an interview with Millennium's chief scientific officer. While the press release was careful to use the scientific terminology "metabolic disorders," the science officer spoke of the "fat burning" properties of the drug.

"Burning fat" is a major preoccupation with the media and their public. It was a savvy ploy by the scientific officer to evoke such language, even if he did so unintentionally. No longer simply correcting a metabolic disorder, the potential drug was said to address "the mechanism that allows us to modulate" the burning of fat in the body. The article summed up this position by stating that "the drug…appears to boost fat burning."

A lot was taken for granted in the *WSJ* article. Genetic research appeared powerful. No need to take poisonous toxins that have nasty side effects, because altering genes was just science's way of correcting what Mother Nature has messed up.

The development of genomically derived drugs was marked as "better" because the pharmaceutical company supposedly knew what message *should* have been given in human genes. For example, fixing a "fat gene" assumes that all people *should* have been thin and that nature sent the wrong instructions to those of us who are fat. That "should" is a culturally based assumption, not a biologically proven fact. But it was treated as fact in the article, without any conscious examination.

In all fairness, fixing "the fat gene" was not exactly what Millennium and Abbott wanted to do, and they were careful not to make that claim. No "fat gene" has been proven to exist. What they were selling was the idea that fixing the insulin-regulating enzyme gene will fix fatness.

Metabolism probably has something to do with why some of us can eat anything and never gain an ounce while others of us can eat celery all day long and still gain weight. But this drug was being marketed on the basis of the expressed premise that obesity was not only a disease, but that it was a genetically related metabolic disorder. Further, it was the so-called fat-burning properties of this drug that made it appealing in the public's eye and easy to cover for the media.

The transformation of obesity from a metabolic disorder into a fat-burning imbalance was not the only rhetorical magic taking place. Pay attention, as well, to what happened to the drug itself in the rhetoric of the press release and the rhetoric of the news article.

In the press release, the drug was described as enhancing glucose sensitivity through the regulation of insulin enzyme production. In the news article, the drug was described as controlling a gene for a fat-regulating enzyme. No explanation was offered on how control of insulin regulation controls fat regulation. This gap in the rhetoric was as wide as the 80-million-person discrepancy.

The fact that "fat-burning" properties were emphasized in the subsequent news stories based upon the announcement of Phase I clinical trials on a drug that tinkered with glucose sensitivity is the most telling part of this case. "Fat-burning" is an instantly recognizable cultural metaphor that doesn't really have much scientific support. It is true that the use of calories in the daily function of the body is an expenditure of energy, much like fire expends energy through burning. But the "heat" metaphor pretty much ends there.

The human body turns food into units of energy called calories. Then calories are expended in the maintenance of human internal systems. This is a complex process requiring chemical reactions among the macronutrients (carbohydrates, proteins and fats) we ingest and those chemicals in our bodies that extract the molecules needed and use them to keep the body going. A needed byproduct of these macronutrient reactions is glucose, which is released into the bloodstream.

Glucose is especially important to provide fuel for muscles, including the heart. The body can make glucose from all three macronutrients, but carbohydrates are the easiest to convert because they already have the basic molecules.

Too much glucose in the blood system creates a number of health problems, collectively called diabetes. Too little glucose in the blood system also creates health problems, collectively called hypoglycemia. To ensure that glucose stays at an optimum level, the pancreas secretes two kinds of enzymes: glucagon, which increases glucose, and insulin, which decreases glucose. Only glucose in the blood, not fat or protein, will stimulate the pancreas to produce insulin.

Insulin works by bonding with glucose molecules in the blood and then bonding with organs that need the glucose, allowing energy to get to the parts of the body that need it most. Far from *burning* fat, insulin *uses* fat cells in the blood stream to regulate itself and do its job. A 100 percent fat-free diet would be as dangerous as a 100 percent all-glucose diet.

Type 1 diabetes is the condition in which the pancreas is incapable of making insulin. Type 2 diabetes is the condition in which the pancreas does not make *enough* insulin because the pancreas loses glucose sensitivity and doesn't trigger the release of enough insulin to lower glucose levels.

Since Type 1 diabetics make no natural insulin, they must take shots of insulin to help maintain their glucose levels. Type 2 diabetics can usually regulate their glucose through exercise, which utilizes more glucose in the muscles to keep up with the extra energy expenditure, and through lowering carbohydrate and fat intake. Nowhere in this process is fat burned, and nowhere in the press release or the article about MLN4760 is this process made explicit.

Changes in diet and exercise might result in minor changes in weight, but there is ample evidence that the metabolic health of Type 2 diabetics can be achieved with little or no weight loss. It is the lifestyle changes, not weight loss, that help maintain optimum glucose levels and reduce the complications from Type 2 diabetes.[11]

The Millennium/Abbott press release and subsequent news coverage is a perfect example of how "obesity" remains an elusive term with little scientific meaning. Some people assert that the clinical definition of a Body Mass Index (BMI) of greater that 30 is precise enough. However, the fact that such a definition includes body-builders and people with lots of lean body mass as well as those with higher percentages of body fat reveals the BMI definition as culturally symbolic but too imprecise for good science.

The truth is that obesity is talked about as if it were a disease, a condition, a symptom, a genetic disposition, and a body-type description. The context in which the word is mentioned often determines its meaning.

So is one to assume that the pharmaceutical company science officer was unaware of how insulin works in the body and doesn't know about lifestyle changes that increase insulin and glucose sensitivity? My guess is that the science officer knew exactly how insulin worked, and, if asked, would admit that the term "fat burning" is more metaphorical than scientific.

The metaphor relies as much on our collective anxiety and fear of fat as it does on any particular health benefits. Our fear of fat lies in our fear of ostracism and stigmatization more than it does in a fear of ill health.

Practically every product or service that promises weight loss promises fat burning in some form or another. "Pounds will melt away." "You will burn fat, not lose muscle." "You can lose weight while you sleep with our fat burning formula." "Developing your muscles has fat-burning properties." These stories are told millions of times a day in thousands of venues such as web pages, infomercials, newspaper ads, magazine ads, radio commercials and television commercials. Many of these commercials show "before and after pictures" that are meant to make the fat body look as ugly as possible and the thin body look as appealing as possible.

According to a Federal Trade Commission staff report dated September 2002 called *Weight-Loss Advertising: An Analysis of Current Trends,* 42 percent of the weight loss ads in their sample (taken from 1991 to 2001) included before and after pictures. These pictures were used as testimonials, used to illustrate effects on specific body parts (by showing only the abdomen or the thighs, for example), and used to show a transformation from a fat body to a thin body (usually without being clear as to whether a computer-enhanced image was showing you what the product could do or if time-lapse photography was showing what the product had done).

Illustrated testimonials consistently showed "before" pictures depicting the subject in a "snapshot quality photograph…that incorporates poor posture, neutral facial expression, unkempt hair, unfashionable attire, poor lighting, and washed out skin tones." The "after" pictures depicted subjects through a "brightly lit (sometimes studio portrait quality) pose of a smiling subject in fashionable, often skimpy, attire, shoulders held back, tummy tucked in, with a stylish hair style and carefully applied makeup."

The fat-burning story is a story born out of beauty, not health. The ideal body, according to this story, is fat free, either as slender chic or hard-body tough. No weight-loss ad shows before and after pictures of medical tests, livers, pancreases or hearts.[12] They rely upon words like "burned," "busted," "chiseled," "sculpted," "killer," "mastery" and "melted." These words reveal a hatred of fat.

It is no wonder that even the most "scientific" of studies would resort to such popular rhetoric. It is a powerful way to manipulate a market, put pressure on government agencies, and entice stockholders to invest in research and development.

It is no wonder, then, that I (and many like me) have felt at war with my body fat. In this rhetoric, fat is not part of the body but something horrible, clinging to the real person, waiting to be removed violently so as to ensure it will not come back and kill the person. These ads are encouraging a self-image at war with its own flesh.

Judging from the language these ads usually take, like all good magic acts, the disappearance of fat is death-defying. There are, apparently, no gentle ways to remove fat from one's body. The violent metaphors are abundant, pervasive, and powerful, especially when the message is that being fat is to be hated and is a sign of personal failure.

Cures for fatness always assume fat to be a disease, disorder, or symptom that must be treated whether the cure is obviously false or "scientifically" boosted. But cures are not usually motivated by health alone. The cultural be-lief that fat is ugly is used to promote these cures. Beauty is not separated from health.

The fear of fat, pervasive in our culture, was relied upon by Millennium/Abbott in order to make a profit and by the *WSJ* in order to sell newspapers. Their authors relied upon their audience to be impressed with all things "scien-

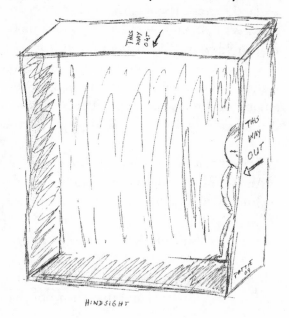

HINDSIGHT

tific" and to be motivated with the cultural imperative to burn fat.

Misdirection of our attention to science hid the motive of prof-it-making behind such announcements. Connecting that science to "burning fat" seals the deal with a double whammy of health and beauty. Smoke, mirrors and our preconceived notions were meant to fool us into seeing things that just weren't there.

Strong cultural and economic interests bond health and beauty together, making it difficult for the average person to separate the two. Because fat is considered ugly and unwanted, patients have demanded that medicine give them a way out, and medicine has responded in ways that keep the spiral of disease and cure perpetually moving. The investments that patients, doctors, researchers, manufacturers and professionals have made in the fat-is-a-disease story make it difficult to burst the 30-to-40-billion-dollar bubble. But there are other costs that need to be considered.

By waging a war on fat, the diet-pharmaceutical industrial com-plex is using people as guinea pigs for dangerous medications and cu-ratives that are killing and maiming people. By waging a war on fat, mass media and advertisers are distorting how young people view eat-ing and exercise. By waging a war on fat, an entire society is wasting resources by spending energy on a war that cannot be won—energy that could be used for better pursuits.

By waging a war on fat, employers, government and educational institutions are ignoring the talents, gifts and humanity of the fattest among us, losing out on what these people have to offer, and con-demning many of them to lives of quiet desperation and loneliness.

Paul Campos, author of *The Obesity Myth,* has aptly said that if Americans want to win the war on obesity, they should just stop fighting it. A cease-fire on fat begins with letting go of the connection between health and beauty. Living free of these entanglements requires a letting go of the medicalization of fatness.

The words "overweight" and "obesity" need to become antiquat-ed, relics of an age gone by. While it is true that fatness and some diseases are correlated and that fat people have higher risk factors for diabetes, some forms of heart disease, and high blood pressure, these correlations are not strong and do not represent a causal relationship.

I am not asking you to forget about health. I am asking you to separate questions of health from questions of beauty.

The rhetoric that turns fat into a disease is rhetoric based in the belief that fat is ugly. There is no scientific basis for the disease called "obesity." It is a metaphorical disease that represents the entire stigma placed upon fat bodies.

Step Three towards a more beautiful you is to talk the talk—and the word is F-A-T, not "obese."

Fat is a description. *Obesity* is a claim; one I believe is a false claim.

I found saying the word "fat" difficult at first. I practiced a lot in cyberspace, but I had a great deal of problem actually saying it without any hint of defensiveness or uneasiness in meat space.

For a while, I said, "I'm unapologetically fat." Eventually, I began to use the word by itself, as a description.

However, as I've been writing this book, when someone has asked, "What is your book about?" I often hesitate and take a deep breath before answering, "It's about the stigmatization placed on fat people."

Step Three to a beautiful you is to talk the talk. Let go of the "O" words (*overweight* and *obesity)* and all the medicalization and fat hatred they represent, and embrace the word "fat."

It can be difficult, but then most liberating things are.

Step #4: Walk the walk.

From the start, our small NAAFA chapter took a confrontational stance with regard to the health professions. We accused them— doctors, psychologists, and public health officials—of concealing and distorting the facts about fat that were contained in their own professional research journals. In doing so, they betrayed us and played into the hands of the multibillion-dollar weight loss industry, which exploits fear of fat and contempt toward fat people as a means to make more money. We asserted that most fat people are fat because of biology, and that the "cure"—dieting—actually causes diseases ranging from heart attacks to eating disorders. We rejected weight loss as a solution to fat people's problems.

Sara Golda Bracha Fishman
activist & founding member of The Fat Underground

In 1988, Michael Weiss wrote a book that

should have changed the way sociologists approached issues of class. It didn't, but it should have.

The *Clustering of America* shared the dirty little secret of how Americans divide themselves into groups. Traditional sociology examined socio-economic status, gender, race and ethnicity as determinants of the kinds of the lifestyles Americans led and the limitations upon life chances for members of those groups. The truth is, according to Weiss and the advertising execs upon whose work Weiss based his book, what Americans have most in common with their neighbors is what they buy.

Buying habits are predictable according to where Americans choose and/or are able to live. Almost since the inception of zip codes and postal codes in North America, advertising executives have targeted markets on the basis of (1) social rank, (2) mobility, (3) race/ ethnicity, (4) family life stage, and (5) housing style. They have as a practical matter connected these characteristics to specific zip or postal codes. One of the most widely used systems, Claritas' PRIZM, has produced 62 clusters that represent groups with a specific combination of characteristics, and these characteristics predict consumption. Advertising agencies pay big bucks to have access to these 62 clusters, and they design their marketing strategies to reflect the assumption that where people chose to live predicts uniquely well what people will buy. "Clustering" concludes that similar individuals live near each other, and pursues this conclusion aggressively.

This may be common sense. What we can afford to rent or buy, the architecture of the buildings in which we live, the characteristics of the neighborhood most certainly would reflect our ability to pay for things and our tastes. But a deeper contemplation of these clusters may reveal some things that should not just be taken for granted, the empirical grounding of clustering notwithstanding.

Marketers often model their approaches to markets as if they were linear. The 62 clusters are meant to tell the marketers the needs of the market; the marketers consequently respond to those needs. Another reading, however, might be that marketers then train those markets to *want* certain products.

Rather than a linear model, one can imagine a spiral effect, with people choosing a neighborhood because of certain tastes and then being educated about what those tastes mean through their mail, tele-marketing, billboards, and so on. They see their neighbors purchasing many of the same things, which they then purchase in an effort to be a part of the neighborhood. Then more advertising responds to those purchases, shoring up the desire to be loyal to those products and their competitors. The push-pull of the spiral effect escalates from there.

Is this predictable? Or is it constructed? No one quite knows who the chicken is and who the egg is and which came first. But the one thing about which everyone agrees is that the "haves" are consuming a lot, and to a lesser extent, almost everyone agrees that they are do-ing so at the expense of the "have-nots" when looked at from a global perspective.

Since 1999, when an explosion of marchers showed up at a regu-lar meeting of the World Trade Organization, protesting what the news media has reduced rhetorically to "globalization," a black cloud of suspicion regarding our consumption has hung over our collective heads. The truth is that long before the street protests at multi-national trade meetings, a growing number of people outside the advertising industry were coming to understand that consumption has become the key battleground for the hearts and minds of people.

Understanding why we consume, in what ways we respond to calls for consumption, and how we construct our selves in relationship to what we consume will help us understand how contemporary Western society works. Such understanding could also help break the spell of consumption as a sustainable approach to economics and reveal the ways in which unchecked consumption is leading to a world of haves, have-nots, and ecological disasters.

Unfortunately, this questioning of consumption has coincided with the so-called war on obesity, and a number of cultural critiques have decided that fatness is the perfect symbol for over-consumption. Fat people have not found many friends among culture jammers, cultural critics and what Juliet B. Schor, author of *The Overspent American,* calls "downshifters." The super-sized McDonald's meal and the super-sized fat person have found themselves coupled in a symbolic indictment of the American lifestyle.

I can remember the first tinge of betrayal I felt when I was listening to an interview on the radio with Frances Moore Lappe, author of *Diet for a Small Planet.*

Moore Lappe's work on democracy, local centers of power and food production have impressed me greatly over the years. I have read several of her books and given money to her organization. In her interview, and, in my opinion, in direct opposition to her understanding of how local systems worked to solve specific problems, she laid out a party line on the troubles of the "epidemic of obesity." Fat Americans were indicative of how overfed and all-consuming our economy had become.

Yep, never mind about the SUVs and 20,000-square-foot houses and poisonous noxious fumes that were hurting the soil, the water and the air. *Fat people* were the problem, or at least, the proof that America had lost her way. I was stunned, but it was just the first in a long series of betrayals I have felt from what I thought were kindred minds to my beliefs about consumption.

Adbusters magazine, a Vancouver-based bi-monthly journal that tries to turn advertising on itself by creating slick ads with socially conscious messages, has received praise from fat activists because of their spoof ads based on Calvin Klein's *Obsession* campaign. One ad shows a thin female figure's abdomen with a toilet in the background, suggesting a purging. Another, entitled "Reality," shows a fairly normal male abdomen (no washboard abs and a bit of a belly) in the same pose as the hard-bodied male model in Calvin Klein's ad.

But *Adbusters* has been fairly typical of the left and reminiscent of my experience with feminists in its treatment of fat bodies. There is an understanding that "too-thin" images are exploitative and mislead audiences, but there is no understanding that fat acceptance means an end to all fat hatred. Larger people are fair game for symbolic images in the magazine.

The most offensive of these symbols is a popular poster showing a distended dark-skinned belly, denoting hunger, juxtaposed to a large light-skinned male belly, implying that it is fat people who are taking food from the mouths of the starving Third World. Ironically, it is Moore Lappe's work that demonstrates the lie behind this poster, as she aptly has shown that enough food is available in the world; it is the politics of distribution that prevent food getting to hungry mouths, not a shortage of food. It is waste, not scarcity, that creates hunger.

Probably the most offensive anti-consumption crusaders using fat bodies to further their cause have been People for the Ethical Treatment of Animals (PETA). It seems that in PETA's politics, animals have rights, but fat people do not.

The National Association for the Advancement of Fat Acceptance (NAAFA) has had conflicts with PETA on more than one occasion. In 2002, PETA pulled a series of billboard ads put up near airports (shortly after Southwest Airlines announced they would be enforcing their "two-seat" requirement for fat travelers) that showed a large man's belly poking out from his T-shirt with the caption "Don't Buy Two Seats, Go

Vegetarian." Within weeks after pulling the fat fliers ad, PETA opened a new campaign with an announcement including the statement that Elvis's fans were inspired not only by his music but his unhealthy life-style, "judging from their own broadening bellies and bottoms."

One NAAFA spokesperson pointed out that the strategy of put-ting on one offensive campaign, waiting for the protest, pulling it, and then following it up with yet another offensive campaign, was suspi-cious. I think it probably could be said to be obvious.

This, of course, is the problem with protests in general. They frequently have the effect of enhancing the publicity of the offensive act. I am quite certain PETA knows exactly what it is doing and has no qualms about using fat people and fat protesters to further its cause.

NAAFA quotes PETA's President Ingrid Newkirk as defending the ad campaigns by saying, "We're not fighting fat people, but we are fighting fat. Used to be you would look around, and there might be one fat person. And now you look around, and the floor is shaking. I think they're going to have to reinforce more than the cockpit."[13]

The thinking seems to be "Why not jump on the media band-wagon?" The war on obesity gets news coverage these days second only to whatever crisis is happening in the Middle East on a given day.

I do not mean to be glib. I only point out that if Vulcans were monitoring CNN broadcasts to determine what was happening on Earth, they would believe the only conflict on the planet was in the Middle East, and the only problem Earthlings were having was getting fatter. So PETA's strategy of tying its wagon to one of the Big Two seems savvy, if you are willing to discount its endorsement of the prejudice underlying the "war on obesity."

A 2004 visit to PETA's website shows they haven't changed much in two years. Their "milk sucks" campaign has made obesity central to their call for the end of consuming dairy products. It has not done so kindly. I found two particularly outrageous examples on the site—one a "Mother's Day" e-card and the other an animated cartoon of "Chubby Charlie."

The e-card can be e-mailed to anyone you want for free. It opens with a panel that spells out MOTHER, each letter representing a message supposedly addressed to Mom:

> M is for the cow's milk that you gave me.
> O is for the obesity it brought
> T is for the tummy cramps that plagued me
> H is for the heart disease I've got
> E is for the earaches that I suffered
> R is for the runny nose of snot
> Put them all together, they spell "MOTHER"
> The milk you fed me sure gave me a lot!

Click on "next" to "open" the virtual greeting card and you see a fat male. It is difficult to decide if he is a man or a boy because on one hand, he is wearing a beanie, but on the other hand, he has a mature face.

He is wearing juvenile clothes that are too small for him. His large belly remains uncovered by his small T-shirt. His shorts are also too small and are torn, with his thighs squeezed into them like a balloon pinched off at the knees. His swollen calves are also ballooned and tucked into too tight shoes. He is pimply faced, snot is running from his nose, and he is drinking milk through a straw. The caption reads: "Would it have killed you to breast-feed?"

The third panel reads:

> Research links the consumption of dairy products to a host of diseases and chronic conditions. Infants fed cow's milk-based formula are more likely to suffer from painful cramps of colic than babies fed soy-based formula or breast-fed. For toddlers and older children, milk is the number one source of allergies, and studies link milk with ear infections, insulin-dependent juvenile-onset (Type 1) diabetes, asthma, recurrent bronchitis, mucus production, flatulence, constipation and other ailments. A lifetime of consumer fat-laden dairy products contributes to heart disease. America's number one killer, as well as the obesity that's sweeping the nation. Breast milk is the best food for infants. If breast-feeding isn't pos-

sible, a soy-based formula made specifically for newborns meets nutritional needs without causing health problems. For children older than 12 months, fortified soy or rice milk is a healthy choice.

These assertions about the connection of milk and fatness are made with no documentation. The card relies upon a tired, stereotypical vision of fatness as lazy, ugly and sickly. The juvenile aspects of the image tap into the current "do it for the children" mentality that the war on fat has taken lately.

I also find the "blame mother" aspect of the card offensive as well. Actually, to be honest, I am not so much offended as bored. The card was so stereotypical and so worn that I find it difficult to believe anyone would be amused or shocked.

Expecting an e-card to document its claims might be asking a bit much. The milksucks.com web site run by PETA actually does offer documentation, but only after you get to see a grotesque cartoon called "Chubby Charlie."

Upon clicking on the cartoon button, the first panel you see briefly (I had to watch the cartoon about six times to be able to read the entire message) says, "Eat fat and you'll be fat. Be kind to animals and your butt and gut by avoiding fattening dairy products."

The panel transitions into a panel with an animated fat man laid out on a chair, pouring milk down his throat until it is coming out his ears and filling the room, stopping right before it is high enough to drown him. Mucus is pouring from nose, ears, & eyes. Several milk cartons are lying on the ground at his feet. Sucking noises can be heard as the room fills up with milk. Like the male in the Mother's Day card, "Chubby Charlie" is wearing juvenile clothes that are too small for him.

There is a button for "more information" that leads to the same unnamed "medical experts" stating that "300,000 Americans die from weight-related illnesses every year, making fat the country's number-two cause of preventable deaths." There are also pithy statements like: "Dump the meat and dairy, and you're likely to lose those unwanted pounds!" and "You'll look fabulous and have loads of energy too."

PETA's agenda with its "Got Obesity" (a play on the "Got Milk" ads put out by the dairy industry) is to make milk drinking as ugly an experience as possible. What could be uglier than fat people? But PETA is only tapping into a pervasive cultural attitude about fatness and beauty. Apparently they have decided it is okay to foster prejudice as long as the prejudices are popular ones.

These images are blatantly bigoted. It is interesting, for example, that PETA uses images of white men in these campaigns. The public would probably not tolerate a person of color or a woman depicted in such a manner. Depicting a person of color as shiftless, lazy and over-indulgent would have invited more than NAAFA's attention. But the bigotry is made okay because of the "health concern" for fat people.

In its own view, apparently, PETA is only educating a fat public about the evils of consumption of animal fat. It does not question the "epidemic" or the connection of fat to eating, because it is convenient to use the epidemic rhetoric to further the animal rights cause.

The Fat Underground understood as early as the 1970s that confronting the belief that "fat is unhealthy" is a central piece to changing attitudes about fat people. As long as the health excuse exists fat bigotry will be okay, because those practicing bigotry can state with assurance that they are only concerned about fat people's health.

Research and curative interests are supported by the bigotry of images and ideas that put fat people at the center of the global social justice movement's desire to confront Americans with over-consumption. Claims about epidemics and ill health give the anti-consumption crowd something to hook into that gets them attention from a media obsessed with fatness. In the middle stands the fat person, stigmatized and, often, violated, simply because of the way they look.

The sad irony is that the wasted efforts people make each year to get thin and/or stay thin are themselves a rich story of over-consumption. If anti-consumption activists were not so blinded by the culture pulled over their eyes, they would find fat activists a fine ally. What is more quintessential American consumerism than the wasting of resources year after year on products that do not work?

Landfills are full of exercise machines, plastic bottles from diet pills, and other weight loss gadgetry that have been thrown out while similar gadgetry and supplements have been bought for yet another try at weight loss. Millions of dollars are spent every year on health club memberships that are never used because instead of simply enjoying movement, we get discouraged when we cannot lose weight. Hospitals in the US are using valuable time and space to cut up perfectly normal stomachs while millions of people in the world have no medical care available at all.

Newspapers and television stations waste time and effort on the "Obesity Summit" of 2004 and similar events while giving virtually no time at all to the ravishes of starvation, disease, war, and genocide that plague a good part of the globe. Talents and skills are wasted on solving a non-existent problem, "obesity," when that brainpower could be used for curing AIDS or exploring Mars.

That doesn't even begin to count the number of fat people who have been tossed out of society even though they have much to offer. Bigotry is costly in both economic and social terms.

In their book *White Racism,* Joe R. Feagin and Hernan Vera outline the material, moral and psychic costs of racism. Many books have been written about the costs of racism to people of color. Feagin and Vera sought to assess the costs of white bigotry for white people.

I found this approach enlightening because so many people who seek to change a stigma do so by concentrating on helping the stigmatized person cope with their lot in life (the stigmatized person often being forced, ridiculously enough, to accept this "help" by largely assuming quietly the subservient role). Bigotry is a problem because one person is mounting an attack on another person. The responsibility to stop the attack is up to the person making the attack, not the person under attack.

It is the person practicing bigotry who needs to change. If it is the responsibility of the person under attack to deal with bigotry instead of the person making the attack, a person engaged in bigoted behavior would be exonerated for his or her behavior. Such an approach to stigma would allow the bigoted strategy to be an optimal strategy, with little consequence to the attacker.

Feagin and Vera suggested that white racism stems from a breakdown in empathy across color lines, and that such a lack of empathy has consequences for all involved:

> Empathy is an essential component of human social life. It tells us that a child's cry means discomfort or hunger or allows us to relate pleasure to a smile and pain to a lament. Empathy permits us to come together and communicate, and it requires significant personal effort. Most importantly for our arguments here, empathy is essential for the resolution of racial oppression and conflict. Empathy at the individual level is essential for real equality at the societal level. Of course, a condition of unreserved empathy would make social life impossibly intense, and a totally empathetic person would find it impossible to hear or watch the evening news. Life in society is made possible by empathy but also by its selective control. Racist thinking is one of this society's ideological systems that fosters a selective expression of empathy. However, in contrast to other empathy control systems, racist thinking is unhealthy for black and white individuals and extraordinarily wasteful for the larger society.

I have discussed the parallels of racism and fat hatred in public forums and have received a heavy scolding for "equating" the two. There is no equating what fat people have gone through with the troubled history of the Black holocaust, the Native American genocide, or the criminalization of homosexuality. That is because there is no equating any of these systems of bigotry with each other.

The experiences of stigmatized peoples are different because of culture, economics, sociology and history. But lack of empathy on the part of those practicing bigotry is a common element to stigmatization. Deciding that some human beings are worthless simply on the basis of how they look or how their bodies measure up to other bodies is morally repugnant and socially wasteful.

Walking the walk is about confronting fat bigotry wherever it

Forming Three Wise Twins, LLC and The Ample Traveler in 2004 with my brother, Stephen Thomas, and husband, Carl Wilkerson.

Photo 2004
Stephen Thomas

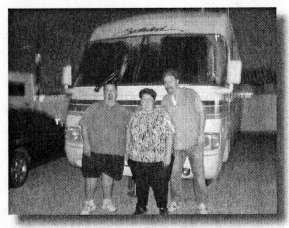

rears its ugly head.

I spoke earlier about beauty and finding beauty in human beings where we can. I asserted that finding beauty is not about pretending that something is beautiful when it is not. It is not "beauty within" and it is not "everything is beautiful in its own way." Bigotry is ugly.

I care deeply about cruelty to animals. I believe wholeheartedly that human beings are far too species-centered in their experiences. I care deeply about the Earth. I am happiest in the forest, and I don't want to see any more forests die. I care deeply about the rate of consumption of North Americans and the impact that has on animals, forests, air, sky, water and earth.

I am not the best at working towards solutions for these problems, nor am I the worst offender. I leave a lighter footprint on the earth than most North Americans, and a heavier one than most of the world.

I do not have all the answers. But I do know one thing deep in my big, fat gut: "Curing obesity" will not solve any of these problems.

The diet-pharmaceutical industrial complex is part of the over-consumption problem. Making fat people the scapegoat is wasting precious time and resources that could be directed towards rethinking consumption and economics.

It is not my job to be the scapegoat. It is not my place to act as poster girl for causes. It is not my responsibility to stop fat bigotry. However, it is my lot in life to deal with the consequences of the symbolic and real violence placed upon fat people every single day.

Walking the walk to a more beautiful me is learning what is my fault and what is not. Walking the walk includes walking away from fat bigotry, not tolerating it in order to be regarded as a nice person. As the great poet laureate and lecturer Audre Lorde is often quoted, "Your silence will not protect you."

Walking the walk means confrontation, anger, unpleasantness and ugliness. Fat is not ugly, but fat hatred is. To pretend it is just a misunderstanding or that if I'm nice enough people who hate fat will not hate me is to miss a really important point. Fat bigotry is about hating people like me.

I am not talking about drawing a line in the sand and choosing up sides. People are not born bigots, and while some of them seem to be consumed with bigotry, most people who do bigoted things are not solely bigots.

Most people who hate fat are capable of love, capable of empathy, and capable of changing their minds. But every time I allow a joke to be made at my expense, every time I back out of a fight because I don't want to be seen as the bitchy fat woman, every time I tone down my anger so I won't get in trouble, I make it more difficult to find the beauty in myself.

This has been a hard lesson for me to learn, and I would be lying if I led others to believe that I have learned this solidly and without fail.

Fat hatred is real. It means that there are people who will think you are ugly just because you are fat. Walking the walk means living life even though those people exist.

Walking the walk means never knowing whether a look, a criticism, a rejection, or a laugh is aimed at you because you are fat.

Walking the walk means being bold and sassy, because being meek and mild is ineffective in a world that judges you by how you look rather than by what you do.

Walking the walk means questioning everything over and over again.

Walking the walk means finding empathy where you can, and

appreciating those people in your life who know your pain.

Walking the walk means becoming stronger for having been tested by fire.

Walking the walk means that at the core of being beautiful is being angry over the injustice, the waste, and the suffering that is fat hatred.

> ## *Step #5: Love the skin you're in.*
>
> *Each twist of fate may have its interpretation, but it also has its beauty...Looking for the acorn affects how we see each other and ourselves, letting us find some beauty in what we see and so love what we see. Thereby we may come to terms with the oddities of human character and the claims of its calling.*
>
>
>
> James Hillman
> psychologist, philosopher & author of *The Soul's Code*
>
>

There are many ways to examine human experience.

Advertisers and media producers would have you believe that human experience is about the products you buy and the products you become. Their ideal of human experience is to leave people forever dissatisfied with their selves, forever longing.

Not long ago, on Big Fat Blog (a website devoted to examining current affairs and fat issues), I became engaged in a discussion about why I felt some pain when I heard about other people trying to lose weight. After all, wasn't it a personal decision?

This is a difficult question to answer. On one hand, I believe telling people what to do with their bodies is the ultimate in limitation of the freedom of individuals. I abhor the kinds of regulations that exist to prevent people from living freely within their own skin. I know human beings have to find ways to coexist in social groups, but I also know that the more regulations of bodies that occur, the more likely it will be that individual freedom will be sacrificed to support the more powerful interests within the group, usually to the detriment not only of the individuals in the group, but to the group itself.

Thus, to make a statement like "your wanting to lose weight leads to my oppression" is an incredibly problematic statement. If people want to have plastic surgery, stomach amputation surgery, have bands wrapped around their stomachs, have plastic bags of saline inserted into their stomachs, eat no fat, eat or drink too much protein, never eat carbs again, report their weight to a counselor or group every week, write down every activity they do, write down every bite they eat, write down the nutritional qualities of everything they eat, exercise until they drop, take pills that make them speed, throw up after every meal, or never eat a blessed thing again, they should be able to do so if they are doing so freely and are of the age to make such decisions. It really is none of my business on a certain level.

On the other hand, every single one of the above activities is dependent upon a portrayal of my body or a body similar to mine as unacceptable. In order to motivate people to do every one of those activities, businesses, medical people, public health officials, politicians, fitness instructors, and pharmaceutical companies have demonized bodies like mine.

As much as those decisions are personal, they are based on an understanding of fatness that asserts that someone who looks like me is stupid, lazy, over-indulgent, and greedy. I don't object to the activities. I object to the demonization.

Frankly, given the current cultural climate, I also question if anyone can freely choose to lose weight. How can anyone know he or she has made a free decision to lose weight in the midst of constant daily bombardments of messages to do so? Since few successful long-term weight-loss strategies are available, one wonders exactly what is being chosen.

The question of choice is a complex question. Choice implies options, freedom and knowledge. Being free to decide what is best for one's body means being able to understand one's body as something distinct from other bodies. Making an informed decision requires access to good sources of knowledge.

In the current climate, *choosing* to try to lose weight may be a misnomer. The stigma fat people face ensures that trying to lose weight can never be purely a personal choice.

Trying to lose weight is usually the only strategy suggested. Trying to lose weight is regarded as the optimal strategy for all fat people. Trying to lose weight is often pushed with little information regarding the hazards of the methods available. Trying to lose weight complies with cultural pressure.

This can be seen when one considers the opposite "choice." A fat person not trying to lose weight is regarded as lazy, lacking "willpower" or "giving up." A choice is not a choice if there is only one possibility.

Over the years, medicine has abused its power in many ways. During the late 1960s and early 1970s, a women's health movement emerged that demanded a simple, yet effective, procedure that would, if followed as outlined, ensure that health care professionals would not abuse their power. That simple procedure is called *informed consent.* This is a powerful counter to medical authority, though it is often ignored or glossed over in the doctor-patient encounter.

Basically, it is the law in most states that a doctor or other medical professional has to tell you the exact nature of your condition, how certain medical professionals can be regarding both the diagnosis and the prognosis of your condition, the treatments available to address your condition, the risks involved in not treating the condition, the risks involved in the various treatments you are offered, and the possibility of seeking out second or third medical opinions. If the medical professional does not give a patient this information, or does not take the time to ensure that the patient understands this information, and something goes wrong, the medical professional is liable for malpractice.

In high-risk medicine, these procedures are followed to the letter. My experience has been that oncologists and anesthesiologists are more forthcoming than family physicians. My experience has also been that public health physicians and clinics frequently ignore informed consent procedures because they believe their clientele will not understand the procedures being offered. So, I am not claiming in any way, shape or form that informed consent has solved the age-old power imbalance that inherently exists in doctor-patient relationships.

Having said that, I think informed consent is extremely important to fat people, and it resolves the public/personal question quite nicely.

I have been privy to a number of weight loss surgery procedures among friends and colleagues over the years. I probably know at least

15 women who have had the surgery in one form or another. Even though weight loss surgery has made a comeback in recent years as a treatment of choice, it has actually been around in some form or another for quite some time. I know of two cases that illustrate the question of informed consent quite well.

One woman was told by her doctor that her inability to conceive was due to the fact that she weighed over 300 pounds. She was given "before" and "after" pictures of successful weight loss of other patients. She was told that the risks for the surgery were minimal. She was encouraged to have the surgery before she received an answer from her insurance company regarding coverage, and told she could make payments if they refused to pay for the surgery.

She had several family members who had researched the surgery and were worried she was not a good candidate. She was diabetic and her diabetes was not under control. Her doctor made no mention of the complications that could ensue from having surgery and uncontrolled diabetes. When her family members tried to bring up their concerns, the doctor refused to discuss the matter and said the woman would be better off weighing less. He did not disclose any research supporting this claim, and concentrated almost exclusively on looks rather than health when describing the outcomes of the surgery.

The young woman had the surgery. She had severe complications from the surgery. Her insurance refused to cover the costs of the surgery. She lost her job because she missed so much work recovering from the complications. She lost her insurance because she lost her job, which made getting her diabetes under control even more difficult.

She did not lose weight. She did not curb her consumption of food and, because of her poverty status, she frequently ate highly processed foods that she almost always threw up.

I do not know the outcome of her condition, as I lost touch with her family about a year after her surgery. I do know that during that year, she became progressively sicker and more dependent on her family. I do know that she presented at an emergency room several times due to problems with her diabetes, and was turned away and sent to the weight loss surgeon for followup because no one at the hospital wanted to treat her; no one was sure what portion of her post-surgical condition had resulted from diabetes and what portion had resulted from complications from the surgery.

Another woman I knew had a completely different experience. She spent at least three years researching weight loss surgery. She understood the differences between surgeries and the various risks each type of surgery involved. She interviewed a number of doctors. She attended groups of people who either had had the surgery or were waiting for the surgery. She discussed openly with medical professionals, counselors and friends the reasons to do the surgery and reasons not to do the surgery. If a doctor or nurse pressured her on a point rather than answer her questions, she did not return to them. She wanted answers, and she was not tolerant of brush-offs.

She chose to have the surgery, her decision having been "informed" by any reasonable standard.

I don't agree with her decision. I would have made a different one, personally. However, I totally respect her decision. It was one of the most informed consents of which I've been aware. I made my views on weight loss surgery known during her information-seeking process, and she listened respectfully and considered my opinions.

She had no illusions of being a supermodel when the surgery was finished. She knew why she wanted to do it and what she wanted to accomplish.

The outcome of the surgery, at least in the short term, was positive. Her health has improved. There are those who believe her health improved because she lost weight. I think her health improved because she began to exercise regularly and reorganized her life to minimize stress. That is a matter of debate.

When I think about the experience of these two women, I see the problem with obesity medicine in a nutshell. Fat people who are good medical consumers are rare. The first woman didn't have the education or the financial resources available to the second woman. That made her vulnerable. Since fat women frequently are discriminated against in the workplace, there are more fat women in the first woman's position than in the second. Obesity research, obesity treatment, and obesity social claims do not happen in a social vacuum.

Weight loss surgery is not the only "treatment" modality that lacks good informed consent. Fast track drugs and duplicitous over-the-counter potions have destroyed the health of many fat people as well. I am amazed, now that I know what I know about weight loss methods, that I'm still alive and kicking and that my health is improving as I age.

I tried a number of things, ingested a number of substances and used a number of dangerous gadgets in the name of losing weight. Then one day, driving home from a Take Off Pounds Sensibly (TOPS) meeting around the turn of the millennium, I came to an important realization. My body simply would not lose weight without some drastic and dangerous method. I was exercising daily, eating sensibly, and attending my weekly meetings, and I was neither gaining nor losing weight.

I came to the end of the road on weight loss and, like an alcoholic who hits bottom, I came to a startling and life-changing realization. I have no control over what my body weighs.

I have told many stories about my body over the years. I have told the story about rape and molestation causing me to put a cushion of protective fat on my body. I have told the story of stressful relationships and work situations causing me to overeat. I have told the story of a

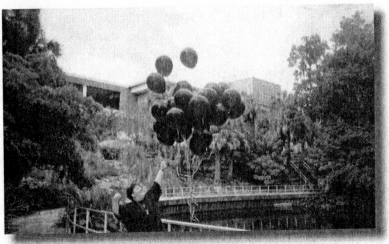

Turning 40 and letting go…

Photo 1997 Carl Wilkerson

weak-minded, weak-willed woman who can't resist chocolate. I have told the story of an emotionally disturbed person who turned to food to comfort her. I have told the story of an ostracized geek who gained weight because she was the ugly duckling.

I've told success stories about my body as well. I lost 80 pounds because I changed my eating habits and exercised more. I lost 85 pounds because I drank a miracle concoction that "burned away" my ugly fat. I lost 130 pounds because I shed my emotional and personal inhibitions (along with my first marriage) and became my true self.

I've told so many stories about my body that I am hesitant to call the "on the road home from TOPS" story the final word, but in a way it has stuck more than any other story has. Since that day on the way home I gave up dieting in all its forms. I stopped weighing myself and I don't let doctors weigh me. When I've had to be weighed (and there are some legitimate reasons to be weighed, such as a lung capacity test or to assess accurate dosage on medications), I stand backwards on the scale and tell the nurse to keep it to herself.

On the road home from TOPS, I asked a simple question: "What if I am just going to be fat the rest of my life and there is nothing I can do about it?" My answer was, "Well, I'd just better learn to be comfortable in my own skin."

That has turned out to be a pretty tall order. I am bombarded daily with messages that tell me I should not be comfortable at all. I often *am* not comfortable. In fact, due to lupus and fibromyalgia, I am frequently in pain. Separating that pain from fatness is a difficult job to do.

But I also found that not dieting has given me a lot of free time. In the years since I stopped trying to lose weight I have written a dissertation, and I have received a Ph.D. I have been involved with several research projects, written numerous research reports, and presented at conferences. I have traveled across Canada and the United States several times, including a fabulous trip to the Yukon Territory. I have co-produced 30 episodes of an Internet radio show and 50 episodes of a weekly radio documentary show. I have learned how to edit digital film and have co-directed and co-produced six short videos, including a 24-minute documentary. Oh yeah, and I have written this book about being fat.

I have had time to make friends on the Net and in meat space. I have had time to play with my cat. I have had time to deepen my love and my commitment to my partner in life as well as business, my husband, Carl Wilkerson.

Pursuing all of these things has made me much more comfortable in my own skin.

I have also become stronger physically as well as emotionally. In the past year, I have taken up weight training again. Exercising simply for the sake of moving my body has been a thrill for me I never had during all those miles of jogging I did over the years. Despite the limits of arthritis and coping with a chronic, incurable disease, I feel healthier and more content than I ever have before.

Four years ago from the date I am writing this, I was 43 years old and I thought my youth had passed. I will turn 47 later this year and I feel younger than I did at 37. At the risk of sounding like a weight loss commercial, I have to say that *not* dieting has saved my life and my well-being.

Having said all that, on the outside I probably appear disabled at times. I occasionally have to use a cane to get around. I have bad days when I can't get out of bed. I have to be careful about being exposed to germs, sunshine and bad food, because I can have lupus flareups if I'm not careful. I take a multitude of pills every day, including vitamins, herbs and prescription drugs, though not as many as I was taking four years ago.

All of this begs the big question: What is health?

For someone who was bedridden for nearly a year and who copes with pain every day of her life, I define health much differently than I did when I was in my 20s. For me, health is relative.

Since recovering from pneumonia and exercising regularly, I went for over a year without having a cold or flu. That is a very healthy year for me, even though during that year I had several periods of time that I couldn't move around easily. The cold I caught this summer hasn't resulted in an asthma attack and hasn't slowed me down much. That is also healthier than two years ago.

I can tolerate more sunshine than I once could, and I don't have as many rashes or flareups when I'm outside. That is a sign to me that I'm healthier, but it would be a ridiculous measuring stick for someone who didn't have lupus.

Health is relative. In his recent HBO special, comedian Lewis Black listed a number of contradictory statements that health officials announce about what is good and bad for people.

"They don't know anything," he told the audience. "And do you know why they don't know anything? Because each and every one of you is unique. What is good for one person is bad for another!"

That is why we must each learn to be comfortable within our own skin.

Perhaps it is odd that a sociologist would end a critique of health and beauty on such a note. But becoming comfortable in his or her own skin is the task of each individual in his or her relationship to society. Social contexts are not "controls" in the deterministic sense of that word. Different people have more or fewer social resources at their disposal due to how others decide to interact with them.

Fat people's life chances are limited by beliefs that fat is ugly, lazy, unwanted, and unhealthy. But those limits do not mean fat people have no resources at all. We could have more if we were willing to stop dieting and start hanging out with each other. But even with the low prospect of such a fat neutral world blossoming out of the current war on fat, finding beauty in fat people and, indeed, in ourselves, is still a powerful social statement.

It isn't easy, but if you make the decision to find beauty where others don't see it, if you resist the negative messages aimed in your direction, if you talk proudly about fat and forget about "obesity," if you walk away from bigotry and towards empathy and let go of the desire to change your body and instead find comfort under your own skin, you may find a beautiful you waiting to enjoy the world, or, at the very least, survive in it.

*In becoming forcibly and essentially aware
of my mortality, and of what I wished and wanted
for my life, however short it might be,
priorities and omissions became strongly etched
in a merciless light, and what I most regretted
were my silences. Of what had I ever been afraid?
To question or speak as I believe
could have meant pain, or death.
But we all hurt in so many different ways,
all the time, and pain will either change or end.
Death, on the other hand, is the final silence.
And that might be coming quickly, now,
without regard for whether I had ever spoken
what needed to be said, or had only betrayed myself
into small silences, while I planned someday to speak,
or waited for someone else's words. And I began
to recognize a source of power within myself
that comes from the knowledge that while
it is most desirable not to be afraid,
learning to put fear into a perspective
gave me great strength.
I was going to die,
if not sooner then later,
whether or not I had ever spoken myself.
My silences had not protected me.
Your silence will not protect you.*

Andre Lorde
author, poet and lecturer,
upon learning that she had breast cancer.

Building Strength

Three Building Blocks
for a Stronger You

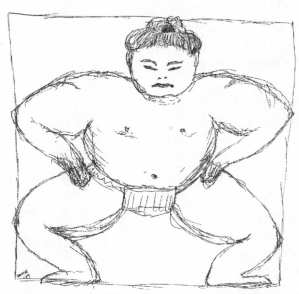

SUMO SPACE

— A Reluctant Warrior

Eyes dart back and forth
Surveying the uncharted territory
Knowing the signs of danger

Fear is something they count on
Fear is something they encourage
Fear keeps the warrior frozen
Fear must be overcome

From where will the attack come?
Will it be the child in the corner,
mimicking her mother's prejudices?
Will it be the diet chatter of the wait staff,
clueless of the implications of their quest for thinness?
Will it be a frontal attack of some well-meaning do-gooder,
who just had a cousin lose weight and wants me to know I can too?

Chairs with arms and small seats
speak of the world where those who don't fit
are not welcomed.
A silent but effective testimony.

Only the most trained warrior eye can see
this tell-tale marking of the ignorant enemy.
"No one told us."

"We can't think of everything."
"We didn't mean it."
"It was other kids."

Chairs without arms hold me in the most welcoming embrace I know.
Chairs without arms say, at least I have a chance.

Pattie Thomas
2004

I have become a reluctant warrior in a war I did not choose and do not particularly want to fight.

I would rather have written a book of poems or some inspirational novel about brave women on a frontier. I'd rather write about the joys of growing older and wiser. I'd rather write about my travels. I would rather tell stories about the interesting jobs I've held or the interesting people I've met. I would rather tell the incredible love story of my life with my soul mate, my husband, Carl Wilkerson.

There are a thousand other things I would rather have written than a book about the stigmatization of fat people. But the central fact of my life to date has been my fat body.

I did not want it to be a central fact. It should have been peripheral. How many people could write a complete book about the implications of having brown eyes? Certainly, no genre about eye color could emerge. Fat bodies should be as neutral as brown eye color. Maybe a few love poems about curves and an erotic scene about the joys of fat loving, but no sociological discussions should have been necessary.

I am a reluctant warrior, but that does not mean I am unwilling to fight. I consider this war on fat a personal attack.

Yes, it is true that most people repeat the statistics and supposed facts with well-meaning concern or, at least, without malice. But the belief that a fat person is ugly, lazy, dirty, undisciplined, unhealthy, and unwanted is nonetheless a belief that I am ugly, lazy, dirty, undisciplined, unhealthy, and unwanted.

This belief has hurt my chances in life. It has made daily relationships difficult. It has made it difficult for me to be gainfully and fully employed in an occupation worthy of my education, skills, abilities and talents. It has meant that I cannot go to public places without fear of harassment and with assurance that space will be made for me.

The war on fat has made my health worse. Being fat has not hurt me as much as has my efforts to rid myself of fat. Years of yo-yo dieting, fighting my own natural tendencies towards being larger, and abusing my body through starvation, laxative and diuretic abuse, drug abuse, and exercising to the point of injury and disability have taken their toll on my body. Since no one really has studied extensively the relationship between different diseases and the various ways of trying to lose weight, I am not able to document this relationship. But I know it exists.

I know that I feel healthier as a fat person than I did as a thin person. I know that since I stopped abusing my body to lose weight and stopped dieting altogether, I have felt better and have experienced better health.

But that does not mean the war on fat has been won by me. Living in the constant stress of never knowing whether I will be ostracized because of my fat takes its toll. I, like most people (especially women) I know, have to work out the calculus of being okay in my own skin on a daily basis.

I still have days where I hate my body for being fat and wish I could be thinner. There are few places I can go, few television stations I can watch, few movies I can enjoy, and few conversations I can have where the belief that my body is not good enough is not part of the experience. With such few positive cultural resources available to draw upon, I am in a constant uphill battle to be okay with myself.

It takes practice to be comfortable under my own skin. It is possible to have more days that are okay, but it is still something I must do proactively. I am bombarded with the contrary message in so many ways that those messages find their way into my brain without my realizing they are there.

No matter how well-meaning it has been, I take the war on fat personally. Of course, I am skeptical of just *how* well-meaning the war has been. A great deal of money is made at the expense of fat people. Little of that money actually goes *to* fat people. Making money in our society is a powerful inducement to continue doing an activity, no matter how ineffective it is when judged by other criteria.

The question before me and fat people like me is, "How do I fight back?" Even a reluctant warrior must be effective in fighting the fight imposed upon her.

In most cultures throughout history, professional soldiers have relied upon a specific discipline and a code of behavior to guide them in their battles. The code is necessary because during a fight you do not want to have to think out the problem, you want to be ready to fight back. The code is important because while your enemy may be predictable to some extent, the surprise attack is always possible. The code is

The Tomb of the Unknown Soldier

In every war there are casualties. Soldiers who die in battle are often held up as symbols of a supreme sacrifice made freely. These symbols are meant to inspire other soldiers and citizens supporting the cause for which the soldiers died. Casualties of the enemy are also symbolic. They represent progress towards victory and an example of the justness of the cause for which one is fighting.

Wars are often measured in death. It is the nature of war. Unfortunately, the war on fat people, often called "the war on obesity," is no different.

Figures like 300,000 or 400,000 or even the newly "revised" estimate of 100,000 deaths a year due to "obesity" are reminiscent of the death counts from Vietnam I used to watch Walter Cronkite give every night on the news when I was a kid. These nameless, faceless figures are designed to sober the viewer into understanding the enormity and seriousness of the

important because without it the fight has no meaning; it is simply raw violence.

With a code, a soldier understands how to fight, with whom she is fighting, and for what she is fighting. Modern warfare is not as explicit about warrior codes as is ancient warfare, but such codes still exist. They exist formally in the chain of command. They exist formally in boot camp training manuals. They exist informally in the camaraderie and group cohesion formed by soldiers before and during combat situations. Having a code makes a soldier strong.

Most fat people are not thought of as being strong. The word "soft" and the word "fat" are often used synonymously to mean "weak." I have had to struggle to remain strong both emotionally and physically with so many negative messages and so few positive messages about my body available to me. However, I have come to believe that it is possible to be a strong person and be a fat person at the same time. In fact, I believe that given what most fat people have endured and overcome,

---

challenge of war.

Many who die on the battlefield are nameless and faceless. That is why many countries have tombs dedicated to those soldiers whose graves were not marked. That is why every Memorial Day the U.S. president puts a wreath on the Tomb of the Unknown Soldier.

Many cultures celebrate the nameless, faceless deaths of enemies by making spectacles of the bodies. Westerners rarely carry body parts around on sticks to demonstrate their victories. Instead, we show the gruesome details of war on television and in magazines. They are spectacles nonetheless, designed to remind the folks back home that it is important to support the cause. They are spectacles designed to celebrate victories, symbolizing the death and destruction of the enemy. Such is the nature of war.

In the war on fat people, I know where such a tomb and

---

most of us *are* strong.

These are truly desperate times for fat people. Being regarded as the number one health problem in America is not a great thing to be. Being labeled as more dangerous to America than terrorism is not a fun thing to be. It has been said that one man's terrorist is another man's freedom fighter, but never in my wildest dreams would I have believed that simply by having the body type that I do, I would be considered a threat to "security" and essentially defined as a symbol of terror.

It is now imperative that fat people remain strong in the face of these assaults. It is my hope that by sharing these three building blocks to strength, those of you who want to join the fight for freedom will be encouraged to do so.

Strengthening our minds, hearts, and bodies in the current cultural and economic climate is a difficult, though necessary task. There are many attempts to weaken our bodies in the name of losing weight.

You don't have to be fat to be a fat warrior. Starving an entire

such a spectacle exist.

On January 29, 2005, Dr. Gunther Von Hagens opened an exhibition called *BODY WORLDS 2* at the California Science Center in Los Angeles. The exhibition encompasses 20,000 square feet and more than 200 plastinated real human body specimens, including more than 20 whole bodies, healthy and unhealthy organs, body parts and slices.

Among the 20 whole bodies is that of a 300-pound man who is displayed in an exhibit entitled *Suicide by Fat—Obesity Revealed.*

Van Hagens may have been well-meaning in his efforts to educate his audiences about health and anatomy. But I have repeatedly said that I have little patience for any "good intentions" when it comes to fat prejudice, and well-intentioned or not, this exhibit is best seen as based more on cultural beliefs about fat than on scientific discovery.

population in the name of health is not just a threat to fat people. What is at stake is nothing less than the freedom for all of us to be what our bodies are meant to be. We are fighting for our beings, our lives.

If you don't think this is a war that results in casualties, then think about the number of people who have died trying to lose weight. Weight loss drugs and schemes have killed hundreds of thousands of people over the years. The development and demise of Meridia, Redux and phen-fen are just the latest in a long list of medical experiments done on fat people.[1] Many more medications are being fast tracked through government approval, and the panic rhetoric will virtually guarantee that dangerous side effects will be ignored in the name of the "war on obesity."

Weight loss surgery is widely reported to have a death rate (number of people who die on the operating table) of 1 in 200 surgeries. A study conducted by David R. Flum of the University of Washington released in October 2003 found that weight loss surgery has a 30-day

---

I raise here the possibility that Von Hagens included the display in question out of his own culturally-induced preconceptions of the nature of fat, and that if he did so, as a "scientist" (i.e., someone who wears the label of "scientist" in his day-to-day life), he of all people should not be allowed to excuse himself for his mistake. Enough controversy exists regarding scientific evidence about the effects of fat on human bodies that at the very least, he should have included multiple points of view regarding fatness and anatomy.

The title of the exhibit alone suggests that Von Hagens has made up his mind regarding fatness. Such a closed-minded stance is hardly in the spirit of scientific inquiry.

"The 'Suicide by Fat—Obesity Revealed' specimen [sic], which shows fat tissue and its relentless, unremitting ability to shorten life by damaging vital organs like the heart and bones..." Von Hagens says on the Science Center's website.

What interested me most in the descriptions of how Von

mortality rate of about 1 in 50. That is, out of every 50 people who have weight loss surgery, one, on average, will die within 30 days of the operation.

There are also a number of postoperative complications that lead to death and disability after the 30-day period. The high demand leading to an astronomical jump in the number of surgeries being performed may have increased the death rate. Several hospitals have decided to no longer offer the surgeries because of the risks involved, and at least one health insurance company no longer covers the surgery because of the risks and complications.

No one knows about the long-term effects of weight loss surgery, because no one has bothered to study them.

Bullying and relentless harassment have contributed to the death tolls as well.[2] A study published in the August 2003 issue of *Archives of Pediatrics & Adolescent Medicine* found that weight-based teasing,

Hagens's plastinated body specimens are constructed is that part of the process is the removal of fat from the corpse. According to the Science Center website's description of the process, "The plastination technique replaces bodily fluids and fat with reactive polymers, such as silicone rubber, epoxy resins, or polyester." The dehydration is necessary because of decomposition. It turns out that fat, like blood, is a living part of the body, one that will continue to decompose after death.

In order to "show" the fat on the 300-pound man, simulated fat was needed. I want to be clear about this. The display is not showing the natural fat that was in this man's body. It is showing Von Hagens' plastinated representation of fat made with reactive polymers.

Von Hagens told Jeannine Stein of the *Los Angeles Times* that he "wanted to include obesity in the first Body Worlds show, which debuted in Osaka, Japan in 1995, but he said it took him 15 years to come up with a polymer that mimicked

harassment, and bullying is widespread among adolescents, and that the victims of this behavior contemplate and attempt suicide more than peers who are not teased. The beatings probably don't help the life expectancy and other health considerations of these targeted children, either. A number of these adolescents reported teasing not only from school peers, but from family members as well.

I cannot help but believe that with the current school initiatives singling out fat kids, we are going to be reading about more and more kids killing themselves. So far, no one seems willing to do anything substantial about fat kids being assaulted, and, indeed, the trend seems to be to blame these kids for the assaults and thus, among other goals, rationalize the denial of remedy.

Fat kids will be ostracized not only by peers and family members, but by teachers, school nurses, and the community, who are often already in the habit of deciding in most specific cases that practically any means to "teach a problem child what he has to learn" is perfectly

---

the thick, whitish look of human fat."

The implications of this exhibit are staggering, and I find myself wanting to write in all directions in reaction to it. But the most overwhelming feeling I have is sadness.

It is incredible how little we (well, some of us) have progressed as human beings. Here is a celebrated exhibition that supposedly is using high technology to impress upon its visitors the wonders of the human body and health. But in the midst of this scientific wonder lies a freak show reminiscent of the many times scientific language and study has been used to reinforce prejudice, misinformation and inhumane treatment. Several similar examples from history come to mind.

Circuses and side shows once featured "savage men" and "monkey men" who were actually Africans paraded before white audiences under captions like "Is it man or beast?" These presentations and representations of people of color were designed to satisfy curiosity about racial differences and

okay. This habit is, as a practical matter, unchecked by any social constraints, unless the child in question has parents who are powerful and willing enough to do something about it. Since fat kids are often regarded as problem children by their parents, it is doubtful that many of them will counteract a school employee's intervention.

Suicide is not the only way in which fat-related bullying results in death. One such example happened close to home in Victoria, British Columbia, Canada, where I lived for four years. Even though I came to the city three years after the tragedy, the beating death of a local teenager remained a dark moment in a small city that prides itself on being one of the most pedestrian friendly and safest places to live in the world.

In November of 1997, 14-year-old Reena Kirk was missing for eight days. People in the Greater Victoria community searched and wondered how it could "happen here." Then her beaten body was

to reassure white onlookers of their own civility and humanity. Such shows were also frequently home for disabled people who were missing limbs or were conjoined twins or mentally challenged. And of course there were the "bearded ladies" and "fat ladies" who were displayed as counter examples to the femininity of the day.

These freak shows often used scientific and educational language to enhance their appeal. "Savage" men were shrouded in Darwinistic terms as "missing links." Disabled "freaks" often told stories about their particular deformity or had a narrator who did so for them. They were often depicted in the side shows as being "able" to do "ordinary" daily activities, as if their having any abilities at all was amazing. The fact that a "fat lady" could walk or talk was equally astounding.

But freak shows were not confined to circuses and road carnivals. The case of the Hottentot Venus is one of the most horrific and dreadful examples of abuse in the name of

found, and eight of her peers were arrested for assault and murder by drowning. Sid Tafler wrote for the Periodical Writers Association of Canada–Victoria Chapter in 1998:

> Reena's curse was her size. Tall and heavy, she towered over other Victoria school girls. And, with deep-set eyes and dark skin, she was considered unattractive, "an ugly," as one boy commented to his teacher when her picture was first flashed across the front pages. In schools full of hundreds of children, she felt alone, yearning for the acceptance and embrace of the peer group, a longing that intensified as the years passed.

It was those peers who were eventually convicted of her murder. But a full understanding of her situation was that she was teased not only on the school grounds, but at home as well. Her social systems

---

science.

Saartje (renamed Sara) Baartman was a young woman who was enslaved in South Africa in the early 1800s and then later taken to Europe by a man named Hendric Cezar, the brother of her slave master. Cezar exhibited Baartman as a freak, claiming she was scientific proof of the inferiority of her race.

Baartman was a member of the Khoi-Khoi people, one of the two oldest groups of people known to inhabit southern Africa. When white settlers began to immigrate into this area, they were intrigued by differences between themselves and the aboriginal bushmen of the area, including their darker skin (which was said to be a pale brown rather than black), their larger buttocks and their ancient language.

The Dutch labeled the Khoi "Hottentots," because of the unusual clicking noises that are part of their language. To the Dutch ear, it seemed that many of their words either sounded like "hot" or "tot."

---

failed her long before she hooked up with the gang that eventually killed her.

The rash of gun violence that has plagued schools across North America has its roots in bullying. Mitchell Johnson killed four girls in Jonesboro, Arkansas in 1998 because he was angry at being constantly harassed about being fat.

Mitchell and Reena remind us that this war on fat is more than a metaphor. It is a reality that fat kids and fat people have to face every single day of their lives. Until something is done about this stigma, it will only get worse.

So when I speak of being a warrior, I do not take this position lightly. I understand that the consequences are grave. I understand that defending myself, and my belief that fatness is simply an adjective, does not guarantee that the stigma placed on fat people will end. The

Cezar played upon many of the speculations among European whites regarding the Khoi, including an assertion that Baartman had "unusually" large genitalia, which "proved" she was not "really" human. This reinforced the Western belief that dark-skinned women were animalistic in their sexuality, and that Khoi women were particularly wild. Hottentots were considered by some Europeans to be a different species than human beings because of their alleged hypersexual nature.

After being sold to an animal trainer in France, Baartman was brought to three prominent French scientists, including Georges Cuvier, at the Museum of Natural History in Paris, for "study." They wanted to see her "Hottentot apron," meaning her genitalia, in order to demonstrate their theory regarding Hottentots. She refused them. A year later she died at the age of 25, from a mysterious disease that some speculate was poison.

After her death, Baartman was autopsied by Cuvier, who made a cast of her body in wax and dissected her remains, preserving her brain and genitalia. The wax body cast and her remains were first displayed at the Museum of Natural History

responsibility of ending fat stigmatization rests on those who practice the bigotry, not on the victims of that bigotry.

So when I speak of being a warrior, I do not expect a victory in the traditional sense in which the term is used. Wars end in "victory" when one side is defeated and the other side is setting the terms. I am a reluctant warrior who wants my enemies to change their minds.

I cannot unilaterally withdraw from this war, because the battle-field consists of ideas that define what my body is and what my body means. But I also cannot unilaterally *end* this war.

Building strength is about enduring this assault. Building strength is about finding the flexibility and agility to face each day. Building strength is about finding balance in a world that is out of kilter when it comes to fatness. Building strength is about carrying my weight well

and then moved to the Museum of Mankind, where they could be seen on display until 1974. (Two excellent sources to learn more about Baartman's story are Barbara Chase-Riboud's historical novel, *Hottentot Venus,* and Zola Maseko's documentary *The Life and Times of Sara Baartman.*)

Baartman's remains were the "property" of the Museum of Mankind and the French government until February 23, 2002, when the French National Assembly voted unanimously to repatriate her to South Africa. On May 6, 2002 Baartman returned home, with the world watching.

The BBC quoted Chief Joseph Little, Chairperson of the National Khoisan Council, regarding her ceremonious home-coming: "The return of her remains marks the end of almost 200 years of degradation, isolation and violation of the dignity of Saartje Baartman. It's good to see that the episode has finally been brought to an end in a dignified manner."

The parallels between the degradation of Baartman's body and that of the unknown fat man displayed in *BODY WORLDS 2* are uncanny. Nearly 200 years after racist scientists sought

in a world that wants me to feel bad about my body.

The time has come to stop the war on fat. The time has come to celebrate body diversity and to build strong bodies in all shapes, sizes and colors.

Everyone will be healthier and happier when we do.

to "prove" their prejudices through self-proclaimed "scientific" means, the faux remains of an unknown soldier in the war on fat people is being displayed so passersby can know that fat people are something other than human.

Fatness is vilified. Fatness is inferior. Fatness is the weakness of a nameless, faceless man who is said to have killed himself by doing the very human act of eating.

The *LA Times* article by Stein describes people viewing the display as "grossed out" and "disgusted." These are the exact responses this display hopes to provoke. In an atmosphere of fat hatred, displaying fat—even simulated fat—and using the term "suicide" plays into the common stigma.

Like the Hottentot Venus, *Suicide by Fat* constitutes a freak show, not science. Like the Hottentot Venus, *Suicide by Fat* relies upon the prejudices and misconceptions of viewers to ensure the message is delivered. Unlike the Hottentot Venus, however, there is no homecoming for this unknown soldier.

I have no idea what this soul hoped to accomplish by donating his body to science. Perhaps his self-hatred was so great that he would be pleased to be displayed as a warning to others about fatness. I know that I have allowed my "before" and "after" images to promote weight loss in the past. I know the self-hatred that would lead to being a poster icon for the cause of fighting fat.

But even if this is what he hoped when he made the decision to make his body a specimen, the display of his body in such a fashion remains a testimony to how incredibly deep and pervasive fat hatred remains in our society. Even if he volunteered for exactly this duty, the display is enthusiastically treating him as if he were less than human.

If you decide to see this travesty, and, as one woman told Stein, you "can't not look" and "want to lose weight really badly" after seeing it, I ask you to consider that this man was more than a fat body.

He loved, he breathed, he might have had children, he might have read books, he might have traveled. In short, he was a human being who lived a life. Try to remember that while you look at the faux fat.

This is not him. This is not even his real body. It is a display. It is a spectacle to simulate what fat means to Von Hagens and the cultural ideas about fat to which Von Hagens is appealing.

This man is a casualty in the war on fat people. It might be more appropriate to lay a wreath at his feet than to gawk at his remains.

His tomb deserves respect and dignity.

Pattie Thomas
March 9, 2005

Building Block #1:

Speak your mind.

On December 6, 1994, with the support of such
corporate sponsors (contributing one million dollars apiece) as Weight
Watchers International, Jenny Craig, Slim-Fast Foods Company, and
Kellogg Company, then-first lady Hillary Clinton and former United
States Surgeon General C. Everett Koop announced a federally funded
nonprofit health initiative called *Shape Up, America!* [3] Unlike other
such efforts by the government that encouraged healthy eating and
exercise, this effort targeted "obesity" as a disease and left room open
for more drastic measures to be used in "helping" people lose weight.

In 1996, after a study was published stating that doctors were not
prescribing diets for their "overweight" patients, Koop announced an
initiative he called "the war on obesity."

Since World War II, when Americans made incredible personal
sacrifices in order to support the war effort in Europe, North Africa
and the Pacific, anyone wishing to mobilize the American public to a
cause has used the word "war" or some similar war imagery to frame
their efforts. So like "the war on poverty," "the war on drugs," "the
war on illiteracy," and "the war on terrorism," the "war on obesity"
was largely intended to be symbolic and motivational. However, like
those similar efforts, this war has turned from something on *behalf* of
a particular population to a war *on* that population. No matter how

well-intended Koop's initial effort, what has ensued has become a war on fat people.

Sociologist Donileen Loseke, in her book *Thinking about Social Problems*, outlines the process by which a person or group of people asserts that a social problem exists and that a particular solution needs to be pursued. Loseke observed that four elements are needed to make a successful social-problems claim.

First, *there must be a specific claim.* This claim must have two elements. It must be a problem that has potential solutions, and it must be something that affects the public good.

Many opponents to specific social-problems claims usually fight such claims on the basis of the latter requirement. That is why, frequently, discussions of social policy reduce down to an argument over whether something is in the realm of public problem or personal responsibility. For example, when arguing the question of unemployment, one side says those who do not have a job are victims of a Federal Reserve policy that seeks a certain percentage of unemployment to manage the economy in the interest of big business. The other side argues that those who do not have a job are simply not trying hard enough and should be more responsible in their efforts.

The second element of social-problems claims is that *someone or some organization is making the claim.* This brings to bear questions of power.

The social-problems claims made by government and business interests are often heard simply because they have access to the avenues by which the public hears claims. Commonly believed experts such as physicians, lawyers, judges, researchers, academics, case workers, consultants, and so forth are often given more attention regarding claims within their fields than those who are affected by a particular policy. Rarely do we see a homeless person leading the way in public discourse about homelessness. Instead, we are more likely to hear the claims of local politicians or downtown businesspersons regarding the impact of homelessness on downtown corridors.

Of course, there are exceptions to this power dynamic, but almost always claims made by the persons who are experiencing the social problem are made by groups rather than individuals. Thus, we have the birth of powerful organizations like Mothers Against Drunk Drivers (MADD) who, when they started, were not persons in powerful positions, but through the efforts of grouping together, have become a powerful voice in public discourse.

Cafe Courage

I walked into the bookstore on the outskirts of Denver looking for the information clerk who was holding a book for me. I was excited to finally be buying the book, and even more excited that the next morning I would be talking to the author, asking him to sign it.

I boldly walked up to the gentleman and said, "I'm Doctor Thomas, and I believe you are holding a book for me."

"Right this way," said the gentleman. He led me to the till at front of the store, where he wanted to know if I was interested in various discounts and newsletters available to me. I smiled, refused all that was offered, and even refused a bag for the book.

Self-assuredly, I took the book to the café to have some tea and cheesecake and begin reading my new acquisition. Then it hit me—that tinge of discomfort down in the pit of my gut that comes from violating a social norm. I pictured myself, the fattest one in the whole bookstore, sitting in the café with a pot of tea and a yummy dessert, proudly reading a book with the "O" word on the cover.

A lengthy conversation began in my head while waiting in line:

You idiot. You are writing a book about being fat that will probably make you a target for all sorts of ridicule, or at least you hope so, because you want people to read it. If you can't sit in this café and proudly read a book with the word "obesity" in the title, then how are you ever going to go around the country and talk about this subject with total strangers? Show some backbone! Buy the damn cheesecake and enjoy it.

Look at all these young people. I am the fattest and oldest thing

The third element identified by Loseke is *the audience*. No claim is made without an audience in mind, and the kind of claim made will vary with that audience and vice versa.

For example, if the social-problems claim considers the solution to

---

here. Besides, shouldn't I be eating something "healthy" in public? If I sit here with a slice of cheesecake, I will be a bad reflection on the book and the movement that the book represents.

Great, so basically you are saying that either (a) you can't eat cheesecake in public because the Fat Nazis say it is bad for you or (b) you can't eat cheesecake in public because it would be bad for the fight against the Fat Nazis. Do you even get how convoluted that is?

Maybe I don't really want cheesecake. Maybe that's why I'm not brave right now, because it isn't something I really want right now.

Are you going to hold the book up while you read so others can see what you are reading?

Maybe…Maybe not.

"May I help you, miss?"

The barista's question jarred me from my internal argument. I grabbed a chocolate-covered graham cracker and asked for a cup of honey ginseng tea. I was exhausted, and I felt like everyone in the two-story, 20,000 square-foot bookstore must have overheard my little argument and was now politely refraining from laughter.

"Did I win that round or not?" I asked myself.

No cheesecake, but as I began to read, I decided to hold *The Obesity Myth* up and just not look around. I didn't want to know if anyone saw me. I wanted to be invisible.

How could holding a book be an act of bravery?

Was this all in my head?

That's the problem with prejudice. I never know.

rely upon changes in law, then the audience in mind will most likely be legislators on some government level. The venue for claims-making will include things like lobbying key law makers, encouraging key groups to write or call key lawmakers, sending experts to testify before key committees, and building coalitions with key interest groups. These claims and audiences are frequently transparent to the public at large, even if public policy is involved.

The final element is *the process of claims-making.* The claim, claims-maker and audience help determine the methodologies used to create a successful social problems claim. These strategies include identifying victims and villains, conducting mass media campaigns, lobbying key interest groups or lawmakers, relying upon science and/or religion to legitimize claims, using celebrity or expert representation, and evoking emotional fervor regarding the issue.

Loseke's observations provide a perfect framework for understanding the war on obesity. The claim is that America is getting fatter and that fatness is a public health issue because being fat causes or contributes to a number of illnesses that could be made better through losing weight.[4] These claims meet both of Loseke's criteria for a social-problems claim.

First, fat is defined as a problem that is solvable. It supposedly is a reliable indicator of ill health and a leading cause of premature death. Losing weight supposedly lowers the risk factor for premature death and ill health. Second, fat is defined as important to the public good. Like cigarette smoking, the claim is that obesity is a public health issue that costs the health care system in time, money and attention. Like cigarette smoking, the claim is that these costs are preventable through changes in behavior and public policy.

The first claims-maker in the war on obesity was C. Everett Koop, a former Surgeon General (someone with prestigious authority). He was an important spokesperson because a social-problems claim regarding health requires a health expert for believability.

Adding further legitimacy to Koop's expertise was the fact that in 1987 Koop refused to do a study ordered by President Reagan to "prove" that abortion had psychological risks for women. What Koop did was review over 200 studies and then refuse to release his 1989 report because he said the studies he reviewed were not done well enough to merit any conclusions. In spite of his well-known political stance against abortion, Koop would not sacrifice scientific research procedures to serve his politics. While his refusal to release the report managed to piss off both sides of the abortion debate, each accusing him of withholding it because of pressure from the other side, he was considered by many to have proven himself to be a scientist beyond reproach.

While Koop will not personally conduct studies or write reports that fail scientific standards, he has no apparent problems using the results of studies and reports that fall short of the standard he set for himself to further a cause for which he is well-funded. To support his "war on obesity," Koop quoted several pieces of research that were questionable because of their methodologies, their conclusions drawn from their own data, and their obviously biased financial ties.

The audience for this social claim is also more complex than one might expect. One would think the audience would be fat people. Isn't the idea here to convince fat people to lose weight in order to be healthier? But that is not the audience to which Koop is speaking, or at least not his only audience. The problem was located in the medical relationship.

It was physicians who were not doing enough to help their fat patients lose weight. It was public health officials who were not doing enough to help a fatter public. It was managed care providers and insurance companies that were not doing enough to pay for the needed medical procedures. It was pharmaceutical companies and health researchers who were not doing enough to find a cure.

This audience serves two purposes in strengthening the social-problems claim being made. First, it makes it a social issue. If the audience were strictly fat people who needed to lose weight, the problem would simply remain a concern of the individual. The fat person alone would be responsible for changing their bodies, and only private interactions with health care professionals would make the process a social one.

Second, this definition of the audience sets the stage for a curative industry. For almost every successful social-problems claim is a group of professionals, manufacturers, and service providers who claim to provide, usually exclusively, the tools to resolve the social problem. Loseke calls this *a social-problems industry.* By claiming that medical professionals, researchers, and funding resources had fallen down on the job, the push to provide grants, create products, and offer new services was increased. The social-problems claim provided the perfect stepping-stone to making money off of people who desired to lose weight.

With the advent of the Bush administration, former Wisconsin governor Tommy Thompson became the U.S. Secretary of Health and Human Services. Thompson was best known for his dismantling of health and welfare in Wisconsin. His appointment was widely regarded as a sign that the new administration had no interest in expanding or

I Could Have Just Died

Audre Lorde once wrote that surviving is one of the most subversive things we can do. "We must always remember, we were not meant to survive."

This evening, while researching for my book, I was reminded again of the Veterans Administration study from the 1960s in which nearly 200 young, healthy fat men were put on a low-calorie, radical diet to see if they could lose weight. They did. They lost an average of 75 pounds. However, after the study ended most of them gained the weight back plus some. Then these perfectly healthy young men lost their health and, in the next few years, one fourth of them died.

As I read about this, suddenly it hit me. Even though I was perfectly healthy before each attempt, I have lost and gained back more than 75 pounds at least three times in my life.

The first time, I was 20 years old. I had just married a youth minister and concerned women from my church kept calling me, asking if I needed money to see a specialist because I was getting so fat. I went to the grandson of one of these women.

promoting public health, and every interest in placing the blame of poverty, ill health, and disability on the victims. It was no surprise, then, that under Thompson, the HHS has changed the government rhetoric regarding fatness to discussions of "personal responsibility."

While it might seem so on the surface, this emphasis on the personal does not conflict with the claim being a social claim. The emphasis is still on the purchasing of gadgetry and services designed to create weight loss. For example, Tommy Thompson gave pedometers to everyone in his office to encourage them to walk 10,000 steps a day.

No one from the government or public health authority has suggested that "personal responsibility" meant the issue was a *private* matter. Quite the opposite; the supposedly worsening problem is

He called himself a biopsychologist or a psychobiologist (I can't remember which). He did hypnosis and biofeedback with me. He had me take huge amounts of vitamins and put me on 800 calories a day. I ran or walked over two miles a day. I lost 85 pounds, which I gained back plus 20 more pounds in less than a year after I moved away and stopped his "therapy."

Two years later, at the age of 22, I went to a bariatric (weight loss) clinic. I drank cider vinegar every morning. For my remaining "meals" I drank liquid protein, which was all the rage. I lost a lot of weight in a hurry, but started getting respiratory infections. My doctor told me to quit the liquid diet. I gained the 80 pounds I lost plus 20 more pounds within six months. But the infections went away.

When I was 29, I went on an 800-calorie-a-day diet, became addicted to speed and Valium, and ran two to four miles every day. I lost 130 pounds, which made me skinnier than I had been since high school. It took me three years to gain it back after I admitted to the drug abuse and quit.

now regarded as impacting health provision for other people. Figures regarding how expensive it is to support fat people due their ill health and their "obvious" refusal to lose weight are bandied about in a number of places, including government reports and public media.

Within the strategies of most social-problems claims lie a villain and a victim. Koop made the fat person a victim, the one who must be saved by those forces in society most qualified and knowledgeable

Of course, there were other times I lost significant amounts of weight, but not 75 pounds. My weight has yo-yoed so much that one friend whom I only see in person every six months or so told me a few years after I stopped dieting, "gee, it's good to finally know what you're going to look like when I see you. You change your body so much, I never knew what to expect."

So why am I crying at the thought of these 50 young, healthy men dying for nothing more than a stupid experiment? Paul Campos, in *The Obesity Myth,* wrote these words about the experiment:

> And what was the reaction to this amazing mortality rate? Were there calls for an investigation of a government experiment that seemed to have killed a significant portion of the healthy young men who took part in it? Hardly. In the years since, this study has been cited more than 200 times in the obesity research literature as evidence for the proposition that 'obesity' is a highly dangerous condition, and that patients suffering from it should therefore accept the risks inherent in potentially dangerous treatments!

I went on my first diet in 1968. They knew then, and they didn't tell me. They had the science then.

Why didn't they tell us? Why is it 2004 before I know about this study and the implications of it?

Suddenly I feel trapped in one of those bad 1950s sci-fi

to do so. Thompson defines fat people as both victim and villain. Fat people trying to lose weight are victims, accepting the grace of their medical saviors. Fat people *not* trying to lose weight are evil villains dragging down a system that affects everyone. A weight loss focus makes a fat person a victim in need of an industry to help save them from the evil adipose. Refusing to lose weight makes a fat person a villain determined to drag the public health system down by risking

movies where the main character finds out that the government knew about the aliens all along and didn't bother to tell anyone because the power structure behind the government had made a deal with the aliens to colonize the Earthlings. My government knew when I was not even 10 years old that dieting might kill me, and it kept that pertinent information to itself.

I am in shock. Like the main character in those sci-fi films, I am aghast and helpless. How do I fight such blatant abuse of power? How can any hero prevail in a world where so little is under our personal control?

All I know to do right now is weep.

Why? Because 50 beautiful young lives were wasted. At the very least, their deaths could have meant something if the results of the experiment had been shared.

Why? Because I know that these 50 were only a few who have died in a long line of experiments that have been done on fat people with or without their knowledge. I know that many more have been maimed, disabled, and made to suffer in the name of weight loss.

Why? Because I know that if those 30 years of yo-yo-ing had killed me, they would have blamed it on "obesity."

Why? Because the daily pain I feel in my joints from lupus is probably directly related to the abuse of 30 years of dieting in order to find some non-existent thin me.

Why?

Because I know I'm still alive and I just realized *again* that I wasn't meant to survive.

the long-term care necessitated by the chronic illnesses losing weight supposedly prevents.

Dividing fat people into these two potential groups has paved the way for more solutions. Now, the corporate player can "motivate" fat people by withholding lucrative jobs, promotions, and benefits, or by insisting upon "curative" behaviors in order to maintain jobs, promotions, and benefits.

Thompson's addition to the war on fat people was to allow the social-problems industry to expand. The Health and Human Resources Healthy America 2010 goals include "workplace" promotion of "healthy lifestyles," including smoking cessation, reduction in alcohol and drug consumption, and the encouragement of weight loss. Costs of such promotions and the rising costs of provision of health insurance benefits have led a number of corporations to consider hiring practices that exclude people who smoke, drink or use recreational drugs, or are fat. The American Civil Liberties Union (ACLU) calls this "lifestyle" discrimination, and is opposed to such practices as a matter of violation of privacy. But these three cases are quite different and more complex than both employers and the ACLU have suggested.

Drug and alcohol abuse on the job clearly affect performance. Random drug testing, mandatory testing of all applicants, and screening against applicants with drug abuse histories was a hot topic in the 1980s. These screenings take workplace behavior and extend it into private life. In other words, instead of dealing with an employee with a problem that has directly affected their work performance or the performance of others, the screening process suggests that *any* use of drugs (and sometimes of alcohol) has the potential to cause problems and should be avoided. I am old enough to remember the protests when these procedures were put in place, and I am old enough to remember that after the initial protests, such screenings became commonplace.

In the 1990s, most places of business and commerce became smoke-free due to concerns about secondhand smoke. A few businesses have refused to hire otherwise qualified applicants who smoke. But not smoking on the job while continuing to smoke in the privacy of one's own home is usually regarded as an acceptable compromise between workplace considerations and the right to privacy. There are no random tests or screenings to see if an employee smokes. In fact, most places of business provide a space where smoking can take place while at work, but away from other employees and/or customers.

Putting "overweight" in the category of "lifestyle" is fraught with problems. This categorization is based upon the simplest view of fatness available. It says people are fat because they eat too much and exercise too little. It says all fat people are at risk for health problems. Since many insurance companies agree with this simple view of fat bodies, companies are compelled to cut benefits costs by excluding heavier employees. This is clearly discrimination, but it is discrimination on the basis of how a person *looks* and not on the basis of what a person *does*.

No one really knows all the factors that create fat bodies. Since the study of fat has always been in the context of fat being bad and something to cure or remove, very few studies have actually asked the more basic question regarding why people get fat. They ask this question only in the context of creating a "cure," and that context makes such studies biased from their inception.

Several twin studies have indicated that a great deal (some reporting up to 80 percent) of the determination of whether someone is fat is based in genetics and not in lifestyle. Many "overweight" and "obese" people are perfectly healthy, do not put a burden on the system, and are capable of doing their jobs with skill and competence. Far from having a problematic "lifestyle," these fat people have a lifestyle compatible with their employment.

Another assumption of the problematic "lifestyle" tag is that weight loss is possible and improves the health of those who lose weight. Since several studies have suggested losing weight, especially through dieting, is actually harmful to health, workplace policies encouraging weight loss leave many fat people between the proverbial rock and a hard place. Statistics are quoted all the time about how much work time is missed by overweight people, but rarely is the question asked as to whether these absences are due to being fat or to trying to get rid of fat. My own experience has been that my efforts to lose weight resulted in far more illness and down time than my decision not to diet or try to lose weight. Your results may vary—but that is the point.

Finally, being overweight rarely endangers the health of other people in the same ways that operating a crane while drunk or second-hand smoke does. I welcome the ACLU's opposition to discrimination against fat people, but as with the benefits some fat people have gained through the American with Disabilities Act, I find the reasoning for protecting fat people's civil liberties to be just as faulty as those who violate their liberties. The rhetoric on both sides of this fence continues to support the social-problems claims made by those who wage the "war on obesity." I also find in the subtext of their argument a belief that the burden of proof lies with those who would protect civil liberties rather than with those who find them inconvenient in a specific cases. Fat people, like all people, should retain human rights, and it should be up to those who would violate those rights to justify their actions.

Included in this ever-expanding social-problems claim about the

What if you are wrong?

An Open Letter to All the Obesity Reformers of the World
originally published November 27, 2002
http://fattypatties.blogspot.com

Dear "Well-Meaning People"—

You quote many scientific studies in your desire to save fat people from the disease called "obesity." But do you really read these studies with a critical mind? Do you really think about how the study is designed, what assumptions are being made, other ways to interpret the results? Numbers are quoted and re-quoted with little understanding of what they mean.

When people think critically about such studies, they are laughed out the door and told that it is dangerous to contemplate fat without understanding obesity. They are told that people could die if the research indicates fat is not a disease.

You are probably dismissing what I am saying right now because you know that I am a fat person. But I ask you to keep an open mind. Examine the fear you are feeling right now. Why

evils of fatness is the assertion that children are victims. Since little success has been had in getting fat adults thinner, the new thinking is that fatness is something that starts in youth. Targeting fat kids will prevent adult fatness, so the thinking goes. Targeting fat kids comes from a number of claims-makers, including pediatricians, childhood psychologists, and school experts who are identifying villains such as fast foods, soda pop, and parental neglect leading to sedentary children eating junk food and never leaving the television or video games.

Children are perfect victims for any social-problems claim. Few people are comfortable arguing against any claim of injury to a child. Debates about childhood obesity rarely doubt the belief that fat children are inherently less healthy than their thinner counterparts, because the cost of doubt is often to be accused of not caring for children and to be ignored as a result. Opposition to these initiatives usually centers around

does it scare you to listen to a fat woman talk about bodies and health? If you really believe you know what is healthy, there is nothing to fear from questioning and critiquing the science. That is how science works. So be a skeptic and read on.

No one really knows much about the human body and fat. Not really. How a study is set up often determines the results. "Obesity" is a medical term, and it was invented before anyone really studied fat. The assumption in medical research has almost always been to treat body fat as a disease and then to research for the effects of the disease and for the cure.

Go ahead, I dare you. Find a scientific study of fat as fat without assuming that fat is a medical condition. A study that asks the question "what is a fat body like?" I don't think you will find much at all.

I'd like for you to consider for one minute that you might be wrong. Maybe obesity isn't a disease at all. Maybe you are trying to cure something that is just natural, just a part of human experience. What if obesity is a myth?

questions of the deleterious effects that singling out certain kids has on their emotional well-being and the likely increase in eating disorders as even more emphasis is put on thinness at even earlier ages.

The maleficent beauty of a "prevention" campaign as a strategy for asserting a social-problems claim is that it is impossible to know how many incidences have been prevented, and this lack of knowledge is often used not to impugn these "prevention" campaigns but to preclude any critical evaluation of them at all. No one really knows

---

People are taking drugs that damage their bodies. People are opting for radical surgeries that at best ruin their social lives and at worst kill them. People are starving themselves because they fear fatness. What if you are wrong? What if you are quoting junk science and espousing life-threatening cures in the name of a prejudice?

This is science, you say? It could never happen that way?

Women's health and African Americans' health have long been damaged by mythical diseases and their very real cures. Medicine and science live in culture. Lots of things have been taken for granted in one generation only to be regarded as junk in a later generation.

Doesn't it seem like an important thing to do before we come up with yet another cure? Where is the money to study fat bodies as something other than a medical object?

A whole bunch of people are experiencing life differently than these so-called medical studies suggest they should. They live long, full lives with little of the illnesses and problems that obesity is supposed to cause. A whole bunch of other people would be healthy if they hadn't tried all the damaging diets, pills, and surgeries that were supposed to give them better health.

Science is supposed to be neutral. It is supposed to change as the empirical observations support or undermine the model. If you are right and obesity is some medical condition that needs a cure, then what are you afraid of? A study that begins

---

how many kids would have gotten fat without a given initiative. What potentially *could* be known is the percentage of overweight children, but determining this number is more problematic than it first appears.

First, human growth happens in spurts and stops. Thus, deciding what a normal 10-year old should weigh is really difficult. When I was 10 years old, I wore a B-cup bra and had already experienced menarche. Most of my peers had not. At five feet tall and 90 pounds, I was the second tallest person in my fifth grade class and probably weighed the

---

with studying fat bodies as the objective (instead of assuming fat as medicalized obesity) would yield confirmation of your beliefs. But you cling to a model that was developed by people with something to sell and then you rebuff the empirical data because it just doesn't fit the model.

So the next time you want to be well-meaning and help a fat friend by laying claim to cures in one form or another, I ask you to consider what you are doing. What is the source of your information? How do you know what you know? How much science have you read thoroughly, critiqued rigorously, and assessed in light of other data? You could be just repeating junk, and junk can kill.

I beg you to be sure before you decide to pass along such unexamined information. If you don't have the time to study it in depth, then shut up and don't repeat advice you hear on television or read in an ad. Otherwise you could be remembered as part of a generation that decided fat people were unworthy of membership in the human race.

Be grateful for your fat friends this Thanksgiving and leave them alone about their health. We know you mean well, but it really does a lot of damage.

Happy Thanksgiving,
Fatty Pattie

---

most, although by adult standards my BMI was normal and maybe even a little sub-normal. Three years later my peers had mostly grown and I had stopped growing taller. I was one of the shortest persons in my class and certainly nowhere near the heaviest, although I had gained 30 pounds and at five foot tall and 120 pounds was considered "overweight" by today's adult standards.

Because of these kinds of differences, competent "experts" have had a hard time deciding how to judge fatness in kids. Average weight and average height measurements are virtually meaningless, even when considering age. Thus, many experts, often desperate for a number to pin on kids in the misguided belief that numbers will be perceived as "objective" measures that indicate changes in health, have decided that the top 15 percent of weights in an age category are "overweight." This is extremely arbitrary, and does not facilitate much in the way of time series comparisons.

It is true that kids in North America are bigger than they used to be. This makes sense given the fact that birth weights are higher because of technology available to detect prenatal problems and prevent premature births and miscarriages. This makes sense given the availability of better nutrition and more food. (Successful social programs such as Head Start and school lunches have fed more poor children at earlier ages.) This makes sense given the health care resources available that help diagnose, prevent, immunize against, and cure diseases that once led to the wasting away of children's bodies. Schools actively participate in providing these resources to their poorer students, meaning that more kids are getting these resources. Instead of celebrating these wonderful signs that Americans have plenty and have successfully and effectively improved the lives of children, Americans are now essentially required to whine and wail about how fat our kids have gotten.

I am aware that the recorded incidence of childhood diabetes is up, though I also know the reason for the increase is a matter of debate and not fact. I am aware of the lack of exercise and cutbacks of school physical education and sports programs. Many kids are experiencing health problems due to the advent and widespread availability of sedentary video games, television, and computers.

I am aware that fast foods and soft drink companies have made inroads into schools, creating customer loyalty among elementary students. I find the cracking down on fat kids to be particularly disturbing in this case. Soft drinks, fast food and junk food are in schools by invitation. One wonders, now that the same school boards are so concerned about the students, if school officials are attempting to distract stakeholders from asking questions about why such soft drinks and junk foods were allowed into the school system in the first place. They invite the products in to shore up funding, and then put programs in place to discourage fat kids from using these products. Perhaps the school districts still want the thin kids to consume these foods and beverages so they can keep their extra monies.

I am also aware that our food is not as nutritious as it once was, and that the leading vegetable consumed by kids under the age of 12 is the french-fried potato. But these things are true for *all* children, whether they are larger or smaller. Working towards increasing playful and enjoyable activity levels, increasing access to more nutritious foods, and fighting the brand-loyalty tactics of *all* products aimed at children are worthy causes. I object to the singling out of fat kids and the belief that reduction in fatness will signal success in these endeavors. It is hostile, it is irresponsible, and it is fallacious. Are we to ignore the health needs of *thin* children in the name of spreading the message that fat is bad?

The "war against obesity" in the past eight years has been extremely effective in getting its message out. Warnings about the dangers of being fat or letting kids get fat are everywhere, in all forms of media.

However, the "war on obesity" has not been successful in its stated objective. Even those most vocal about the evils of fatness will admit that not many people have lost weight and kept it off. But the war rages on, and it seems irrelevant that people can't lose weight without killing, disabling, or endangering themselves.

Given the identity of the claims-makers and the ever-expanding anti-obesity industry, one might think that recognizing the enemy would be quite simple. Every Surgeon General since Koop made his announcement has jumped on the bandwagon. The current administration has made obesity a top domestic issue, effectively diverting attention from other economic and social issues and from escalating difficulties in foreign affairs. HHS Secretary Thompson's record of dismantling public health first in Wisconsin and then the entire country has faded into the background while he makes news frequently pointing to obesity as the nation's number one health problem. The current U.S. Surgeon General, Richard Carmona, has called obesity the most pressing issue in health facing Americans today, in spite of bioterrorism threats, ecological breakdowns, escalating violence, and the fact that the so-called health care system, as well as the health insurance system, is not available to tens of millions of working poor and middle class people.

One wonders if the rhetoric about the costs of obesity to the health care system isn't a clever way to entice people to believe that an effective health care system exists at all. The timing of the *Shape Up, America!* announcement in 1994, as well as the presence of Hillary Clinton at Koop's side, suggests a connection between concentrating on fat people as a health care issue and the failure of the Clinton initiative to provide universal health care insurance.

In 1993–94, the first lady headed an effort to build a coalition and political will to provide health care coverage for all Americans. This effort included a number of public "town meetings" with "real citizens" as well as public hearings with key health care industry players. All of this effort resulted in what several people have called the greatest coalition-building achievement in recent history.

Of course, the punch line is that it wasn't a coalition of people interested in providing universal health care coverage, but rather a coalition of the private financial interests served by keeping health care coverage private and competitive. Historically, health maintenance organizations, health insurance companies, physician organizations, hospitals, and pharmaceutical companies have been at odds with each other, as their interests often conflict. Because of the Clinton initiative, these interests found common ground and built lasting coalitions that made the opposition to universal health care in the United States stronger than ever.

The strength of the coalition of anti-universal health care coverage interests created a political will to find scapegoats for the rising costs of health care other than the inefficient private system. So-called "lifestyle issues" such as smoking and obesity made perfect scapegoats, because the same people who can't afford health care, the working poor, are the ones with the highest prevalence of diseases thought to be connected to these "lifestyle issues."

By 1994, the first lady was blaming "health care deadbeats" for rising costs. Jumping on the anti-obesity bandwagon seems to be consistent with the search for scapegoats, and the timing, at the very least, gives one pause. Of course, as with the "deadbeat" rhetoric, the *Shape Up, America!* campaign concentrated on blaming the poor person rather than addressing any social or economic factors that might be contributing to their health needs.

Meanwhile, the number of Americans who had no health care coverage continued to rise. In addition, the quality of coverage of health insurance and HMOs went down, while the cost of such coverage went up.

By 1997, frustration with the ridiculous extent to which HMOs determine health care was reflected in the movie *As Good As It Gets*. In a now infamous scene, the single mother of a sick boy (played by Helen Hunt) is told that effective treatment for her son's condition is available. Hospital emergency room personnel had told her there was no treatment for her son's condition. It turned out that treatment existed, but was not covered by her insurance plan, so they had withheld it. Upon learning that her son had suffered needlessly for some time, Hunt's character exclaims, "Fucking HMO bastard pieces of shit!" To which the doctor, played by Harold Ramis, responds, "It's okay. Actually, I think it's the technical name."

Insurance executives were supposedly shocked when theatre audiences across the United States cheered and clapped in reaction to the scene. Private health care coverage, it seems, is no guarantee that needed treatment will be available even to those lucky enough to have had coverage at the end of the 20th century.

Public health has not been faring any better. In 2001, a group of public health care officials, including then-Surgeon General David Satcher, discussed openly, in forums like PBS's *NewsHour with Jim Lehrer*, the declining infrastructure of the public health care system in the United States. In October 2001 Senator Bill Frist told a senate committee in charge of looking into how prepared the United States health system was to confront bioterrorism that there were "serious gaps" in public health. Even Tommy Thompson testified before the committee that there was "more we can do, and must do, to strengthen our response."

Rather than turning to his Surgeon General (who, at the time, was David Satcher, a Clinton appointment), on Nov. 1, 2001 Tommy Thompson appointed Donald A. Henderson to be the newly created Director of Public Health Preparedness. This new office was necessary because so many agencies, departments, and law enforcement organizations had pieces of authority in the event of bioterrorism that someone was needed to coordinate any effort to respond. For example, it was the Federal Bureau of Investigation (FBI) and the Federal Emergency Management Agency (FEMA), not the Department of Health and Human Services, that led the investigation into the anthrax deaths in late 2001.

Henderson was a good symbolic choice for coordinating such efforts. From 1966 to 1977, Henderson was in charge of the World Health Organization's efforts to eliminate smallpox throughout the world, and later in the 1990s, he formed Johns Hopkins University's Center on Bio Defense.[5]

Shortly after his appointment, Henderson told PBS's *NewsHour* the biggest problem in public health was "the lack of really good people and adequate numbers at the state and local levels. So many of the health departments have maybe one infectious disease epidemiologist, and that's it."

Providing epidemiological assistance to state public health authorities has resided with the U.S. Public Health Service (USPHS) Commissioned Corps. The USPHS has approximately 6,000 uniformed health care workers directly responsible to the office of the U. S. Surgeon General.

The military image, with "general," "officers" and "uniforms," derives from the history of the public health service, which was formed in 1871 by John Maynard Woodworth to serve merchant seamen working the docks and ships along the eastern seaboard. Woodworth developed the mobile corps of physicians under a military model that remains today. In 1902, after taking on examining the immigrants who arrive at Ellis Island, the Marine Hospital Service became a federally supervised agency and changed its name to "Public Health and Marine Hospital Service." In 1912, it became simply the "United States Public Health Service" and took on the chore of ensuring the health and well-being of the country.

Today, USPHS is overseen by HHS (Tommy Thompson's department) and consists of a wide scattering of federal agencies (10 within HHS) and other departments in the federal government that have some kind of health-related agenda. While the purpose of the USPHS is to ensure health and safety for citizens, the actual work is done through state and local governments. This means that most of these agencies have money and other incentives to offer the states to get on board with the federal agenda, but they do not have much bite when it comes to enforcement. The Centers for Disease Control (CDC), for example, is one USPHS agency that never works in a state unless they are invited by the state's health official. The Surgeon General outlines the priorities of these health concerns and provides the leadership needed to bring state health officials on board with the USPHS agenda. However, the Surgeon General does not direct these agencies. He sends USPHS commissioned officers and staff to assist these agencies and departments.

With the new threats of smallpox and anthrax and the fears about bioterrorism, the USPHS and the Surgeon General have lost some visibility and, therefore, power. In past times of crisis, it was imperative that the Surgeon General be a charismatic and engaging public figure to ensure compliance with the federal agenda. The Surgeon General has to be authoritative because his power comes from cooperation with agencies at the federal and state level. But throughout the bioterrorism crisis, it has been Tommy Thompson who has answered questions regarding preparedness, and it has been agencies like the FBI who have investigated potential crises. Even the task of coordinating health agencies has fallen now to the Director of Public Health Preparedness, not the Surgeon General.

The formation of an official public health system in the United

States has, from its inception, been more of a response than a plan, and its piecemeal organization reflects this reactive nature. On one hand, it has been quite successful in responding to such crises as polio and smallpox. It has been good at dealing with outbreaks of contagious diseases. This has been, in part, because such outbreaks are straightforward within the medical model and, in part, because little profit can be made from such outbreaks. Private interests such as pharmaceutical companies, hospitals, health maintenance organizations, and surgery units make more money from other health considerations than inoculations and antibiotic treatments.[6]

On the other hand, the public perception of health care, including private health care, is that providing health care is becoming more costly, with health care professionals less able to handle long-term care, aging, and chronic conditions. As Senator Frist said so eloquently in 2001, there are gaps. I would add that those gaps include handling the tens of millions of people who do not have access to health care coverage, even public health facilities. The dependency that the United States has on a market-model health care system has left huge gaps in what could be, and is for the richest among us, a superb health care system.

In a way, the threat of bioterrorism has widened those gaps even more. Monies that might have provided better coverage and more efficient delivery of health care needs have been diverted away from public health into preparations for threats that are often more based on fear than reality.

A cynical person might wonder whether suggesting at this particular moment in history that fat people are burdening the public health care system does not provide an extremely convenient patsy at a time when several forces are looking for such a setup. The Surgeon General (now Richard Carmona, a Bush appointment) brings a crisis to the forefront that is seemingly just as "threatening" to the citizenry as the crisis that led to the loss of power for his position. The states have a new way to fund their under-funded and overtaxed public health agencies through potential lawsuits rivaling the tobacco suits of the 1990s. Private, for-profit health care interests have a way to charge more for fewer services, thus making their stockholders happy and finding a way to look good to the government to delay intervention. In addition, all this attention to ineffective dieting methodologies serves to keep Americans from thinking about the tougher questions of universal health care, long-term care, and rising pharmaceutical costs. Jumping on the anti-obesity wagon offers a great deal of perks with little in return.

Surely, the government is a strong candidate as an enemy of fat warriors. Yet their case is undermined by several government agencies which, in spite of the most vocal public health spokespersons saying otherwise, have made reports about the problems with dieting, the importance of emphasizing exercise over weight loss, and the potential damage that stigmatizing fat people can cause.

The Food and Drug Administration (FDA) has cracked down on the most outrageous weight loss claims of late, including encouraging consumers to report bogus claims, pursuing fraud charges against outright lies, and providing guidelines for consumers to use to determine exaggerated and patently false claims. The National Institutes for Health (NIH) have published guidelines for physicians outlining the ways in which fat people have received poor treatment from health care professionals and the ways to be accepting of fat patients, including not pressuring fat patients to lose weight when they have other health problems. The Centers for Disease Control (CDC) has published several reports that suggest dieting is not a good strategy and that losing weight at all costs may be more detrimental to health than a promotion of it.

If not government policy makers, then perhaps health researchers could be the bottleneck. In the June 7, 2004 special issue of *Time,* one of the "Overcoming Obesity in America" feature articles was entitled "The Obesity Warriors." These experts were New York University nutritionist Marion Nestle, Harvard pediatric researcher David Ludwig, Yale psychologist Kelly Brownell, and San Diego State University psychologist James Sallis. There could be many others added to this list.

Author and journalist Laura Fraser, in her book *Losing It,* spoke with a number of obesity researchers, and outlines the ways in which many of them have financial connections to the diet industry that are not often disclosed when they are quoted in popular and academic media. Paul Campos adds some more recent newsmakers to the list in his book *The Obesity Myth,* and further documents the financial and professional interests they have in perpetuating a specific party line without examination or consideration of other points of view:

> As for self-interest, it's fairly clear from their off-the-record comments that some putatively orthodox obesity research-ers are well aware that much of their field is little more than scam masquerading as a science. These researchers, however, are also keenly aware that the economics of the field—a field that is almost wholly funded by the weight loss industry—require that the fundamentally flawed premises at the base of most obesity research should never be examined, let alone criticized.

Making researchers in general the "enemy," however, is under-mined by the fact that there have been, in the past few years, a num-ber of obesity researchers who, because of their research, have changed their minds about fat as a disease. The same kinds of work and experi-mentation, when assessed without the weight loss industry bias, can lead to fat acceptance. So research is both friend and foe, and it is a complicated task to sort through the landscape.

Most of us are not equipped or educated enough in epidemiology and medical research to sit in judgment over the plethora of research that seems to stream into public consciousness on a weekly, if not daily, basis. We should not have to be equipped to do so. Other researchers and medical reporters are supposed to be the watchdogs that level the playing field.

As a social-problems claims industry grows and expands, a class of workers emerge that some sociologists have called *street-level bureaucrats.* These are the workers who most often interact with the victims (and some times villains) of a social-problems claim. It is on their shoulders that the success of a proposed solution rests. In the war on obesity, these are nurses, physicians, nutritionists, kinesiologists, personal trainers, diet gurus, weight loss surgeons, diet book authors, weight-loss group leaders, counselors, and so forth. The street-level bureaucrat would be anyone with whom a fat person might make an appointment to talk about losing weight.

A case could be made that these street-level bureaucrats are the enemy. However, it has been my experience that many of these people, especially those whose living is not contingent directly upon the promotion of weight loss, have already picked up on the fact that most people will not be able to lose weight and maintain the loss for a long period of time. They are willing to work with clients who want to lose weight and guide them in their efforts, but they are often just as willing to take weight loss out of the equation and work with fat clients who just want to be healthy.

One might concede for the sake of argument that, from Tommy Thompson and Richard Carmona all the way down to the leader of my local TOPS chapter, many of these people mean well. They truly believe fat is bad. They truly believe losing weight is good. They truly believe that they are trying to help a group of people desperately fighting for their lives. Perhaps I should not count them as enemies per se. However, "meaning well" does not excuse the damage that has been done by their actions. I may not count them as enemies, but I certainly will not sit by quietly because they had good motives. No matter what their intent, those who perpetuate the bigotry of fat hatred must be confronted.

Perhaps the makers of movies, advertisements, and other forms of media are the enemy. After all, one could argue that the social-problems claim that fat is bad was born both historically and culturally out of a social stigma of fat people. Who perpetuates these stereotypes more vigorously than the entertainment, fashion, and news businesses?

Portrayals of fat people in screenplays and documentaries show supposedly scary, ugly, and/or lazy people. News shows pick up on every fat celebrity's death and sensationalize the event with stories about eating habits and/or exercise habits. Even the death of Orioles pitcher Steve Bechler, which resulted from his attempting to lose weight using the herbal supplement ephedra, led to stories about fat players rather than stories about players who practice anorexic and bulimic behaviors and/or drug misuse in order to stay game-ready. Surely people like the ones who portrayed "Mama" Cass Elliot erroneously as dying from choking on a sandwich instead having a poor heart from drug usage are the enemy of the fat warrior.

Deciding if the media reflects social attitudes or creates social attitudes is an age-old dilemma that makes treating the media as an enemy problematic. One could argue just as easily that books, magazine articles, films, television shows, and radio have been used to promote empathy towards fat people.

Roseanne, the popular sitcom from the late '80s and early '90s, showed fat people having families, having sex, dealing with life, and being human. The cult film and successful Broadway production of *Hairspray* promote a view of a fat kid not only as normal but talented and popular. (The creator of *Hairspray,* John Waters, was once asked why he put fat people in his films. His wonderful response was "because those are the real people I grew up with in Baltimore.") Daniel Pinkwater writes incredibly sensitive, popular children's books with fat kids as heroes. The documentary *Fat Chance,* which told the moving story of a 400-pound Manitoba man's journey to fat acceptance, was produced with the Canadian National Film Board footing the bill. While these media examples are certainly rarer than their opposites, they nonetheless point to how problematic it is to regard the media as the enemy of the fat warrior.

One of my favorite motion pictures is *The Matrix.* As a sociologist, I found the film to be the perfect metaphor for a sociological view of the world: "The matrix is the world pulled over your eyes."

Learning about sociological theory has afforded me a view of the social structures that shape my life and other people's lives in a way that is usually not noticed in everyday life. We do and say things with little thought to how we know what we know or where we learned what we think. Social interactions are often reactions and replications. We often follow certain preset scripts as to what is normal and acceptable in these interactions.

"The matrix" can be seen as a metaphor for this underlying set of rules we all follow without much examination. This *can* be a good thing. If we had to get up every morning and rethink the world, we would never get anything done. Having knowledge of what to expect frees up time and effort for human beings to explore new ideas and new activities.

The metaphor of the matrix, however, also demonstrates what can happen if we follow these rules without ever questioning their validity or revising them over time.

In *The Matrix,* we are told the story of how Morpheus, a leader in the human resistance to a machine-dominated world, finds and teaches Neo, a potential savior of that world, about the structure of the matrix. It is imperative that these resistance fighters enter the machine world of the matrix in order to save the human beings plugged into that world. They are warriors in a struggle with machines determined to keep mankind in the dark about their agenda.

The distinct purpose of these warriors is to save humankind. However, to succeed in saving humankind, they have to plug into the machine world themselves. While in the matrix, they must regard the people they want to save in the general case as the enemy in certain specific cases, because any person within the matrix can be occupied or possessed by an "agent" machine at any given time.

Thus, all those in the matrix who are not warriors have to be regarded as potential machine enemy agents. Until a human being is freed from the matrix, she or he will fight *for* the matrix, either because she or he believes she or he is keeping something secure, or because she or he has been occupied by an agent.

The net result of this situation is that Morpheus, Neo, and the rest of the resistance kill a lot of the people they are trying to save, as Morpheus explains to Neo:

> The matrix is a system, Neo. That system is our enemy. When you're inside, you look around. What do you see? Businessmen. Teachers. Lawyers. Carpenters. The very minds of the people we are trying to save. But until we do, these people are still a part of that system. And that makes them our enemy. You have to understand. Most of these people are not ready to be unplugged. And many of them are so inured, so

hopelessly dependent on the system, that they will fight to protect it.

This may seem cold on the surface, but not if one thinks of the matrix as a world of ideas, with people being the carriers of those ideas. Knowledge *of* the matrix is the only salvation *from* the matrix. Otherwise, being in the matrix feels natural.

Some of the ideas sustaining the matrix originate from the occupants of the matrix because they are ignorant of the matrix. They are well-intended, just trying to do a day's work and get along with other people. Others are unwitting carriers for ideas that they simply replicate without thought. The "agent" occupies them long enough to pass along the idea. Thus, the enemy occupies the ignorant person to replicate misinformation.

Bigoted ideas about fat can occupy anyone, even the most educated among us. The enemy is bigoted ideas.

When I speak of war, I am speaking mostly metaphorically, but stigmatized individuals face more than symbolic violence. Hate crimes are real, and people have been known to kill, maim, rape, and torture in the name of their bigotry. Fat people have faced and continue to face that kind of violence.

Fat kids are bullied physically and emotionally. Fat adults are discriminated against to the point of not having access to the basic physical needs of healthy food, good clothing, good shelter, and basic health care. Fat adults are also unwitting guinea pigs for a number of schemes, pills, and procedures that are designed to produce weight loss but rarely do so effectively or for any length of time. Many fat adults died during these experiments, and others were disabled. Many fat adults who yo-yo dieted (repeatedly lost and regained weight) remain unsure of the effects these experiments have had on their bodies, and they suffer undocumented aftereffects on their health and well-being.

These consequences of the belief that fat people are ugly, lazy, unwanted, and inhuman are not singularly symbolic. However, symbolic violence is not any less important than physical violence. Harassment, discrimination, and stereotyping have real consequences in real people's lives. Symbolic violence shows up in personal interactions, public displays, business transactions, job and school application processes, popular media representations, and daily conversations.

Because the possibility always exists that someone is treating me as a fat person rather than as the individual I am, I live with an underlying and pervasive daily stress. That is the minimum wage of stigmatization. That is why sociologist Erving Goffman described stigma as a spoiled identity—no matter how a stigmatized person presents herself or himself, she or he will be uncertain as to how she or he is being understood. The question of the stigma is always in the background:

> This uncertainty arises not merely from the stigmatized individual's not knowing which of several categories he will be placed in, but also, where the placement is favorable, from his knowing that in their hearts the others may be defining him in terms of his stigma . . . during mixed contacts, the stigmatized individual is likely to feel that he is "on," having to be self-conscious and calculating about the impression he is making, to a degree and in areas of conduct which he assumes others are not.

I have suffered job discrimination even after earning my Ph.D. I have suffered public harassment. I have suffered unsolicited advice about the most personal of matters. I have tolerated jokes made at my expense both in person and from the television. I have spent lonely nights at home because there are places and events at which I know I am not welcome or, at least, there has been no thought to make a space for someone like me. I have been left out of social situations, forgotten, laughed at, teased, and lectured by so-called friends. I have been refused medical care and had medical conditions ignored. These individual acts add up to a stressful life that cannot reach its potential no matter how hard I work and how much I persevere.

Because of the stigma placed upon fat people, every interaction I have is colored by the fact that I am fat. I can never know for sure whether other people are being completely forthright with me. I can never know if the reason for conflict is simple or complex. I can never trust medical advice completely. I can never know if I lost a job or a grant or a client because of my size.

My first job out of graduate school was a horrible job filled with an incredible amount of stress. Making matters worse was the fact that a key member of the staff actively undermined my work. I tried many ways to connect with her. I became so torn up about the tension that I began to keep descriptions of our encounters in my daily journal. The increasing tensions finally escalated into a public confrontation in which our mutual boss took her side in front of guests from another university and other office staff.

I was humiliated. I had spent a lot of money and a lot of time and a lot of effort obtaining an advanced degree only to be treated like the "hired help" one more time.

I left the office holding back tears, and went home to decide how to handle the ambush. To try to make sense of everything, I reviewed my journal. After typing out eight pages of incidences of harassment by this person, I realized that I was indeed being harassed and that many of the comments were related to how slowly I moved and the fact that I took elevators in lieu of stairs. For four months, I had endured this harassment wondering what I was doing to encourage this treatment. I really thought I just wasn't fitting in and that there was something about me that was creating the situation. Was it culture shock? Was I just a novice and it was difficult for me to keep up? Was I just not competent at my job? I truly didn't get the scope or depth of the harassment until I made the list from my journal. I was writing these things down almost daily, yet I remained unclear on the dynamics.

In truth, I still don't know why that staff person did what she did. Did she hate fat people? Well, our boss was fat, but our boss was much more mobile and active than I was. Did she hate disabled people? I had a particularly hard time with lupus and asthma while I was there, and had to use a cane to get around. Did she think I was faking? Did she have someone else in mind for the job and wanted to get rid of me? Was she just crazy or mean-spirited? I've debated her motives in my mind many times.

The truth is that I hated the job. I quit the job, using the staff person's harassment to get out of the contract. I really didn't care afterwards why she did what she did, only that what she did made my life miserable, and I didn't want to be miserable anymore.

Another example of not being sure about the role of fatness is when I first became ill from lupus. Lupus is a difficult condition to diagnose, especially if caught early enough to treat before something potentially fatal happens. Fibromyalgia is similarly elusive because the symptoms mimic so many other conditions, although the diagnostic procedure for fibromyalgia is fairly simple.

After my regular physician ran me through a battery of blood tests, she recommended I go to a rheumatologist to seek a more conclusive diagnosis and treatment. There was only one rheumatologist covered by my HMO, so that is where she sent me. During my first visit, he spent one minute looking over my blood tests and 10 minutes lecturing me on my weight. He did not touch me or examine me in any way. When I tried to talk to him about my feelings and experiences about dieting, he left the room while I was talking. He was so rude that I had to hold back my husband from punching him.

But I made a second appointment, took the aspirin he suggested for the pain I was experiencing, and tried to walk outdoors every day as he suggested.

I got sicker, a lot sicker.

Three weeks later, I returned. I had gained nine pounds. I had done some reading about my symptoms and came armed with questions about fibromyalgia. He told me to go on a diet and get out more, and basically implied that he wasn't sure fibromyalgia was a real thing. He believed that most fibromyalgia pain went away with weight loss and that I should just try harder.

Again, he did not examine my body. In fact, I had the distinct impression that he was afraid to touch me.

I did not make another appointment. I left determined to find another doctor. I called the local chapter of the Arthritis Foundation and asked a bunch of questions about my symptoms. They referred me to another doctor and to a support group. At my first support group meeting, unprompted by me, I heard at least six other women complain about the doctor who had treated me so poorly. Some of them were fat; some were not.

My new doctor examined me completely upon our first meeting. She looked over the bloodwork from earlier in the summer and asked me some specific questions about my symptoms. The diagnosis for fibromyalgia is a simple touch test of 18 points on the body to see if they are painful. If 11 or more of those points are sore, there is a positive diagnosis for fibromyalgia. All 18 points on my body were painful.

It turned out that I also had lupus, and that walking outside was the worst thing I could have been doing because of the troubles people with lupus have with sunshine. It turned out that aspirin is one of the worst pain relievers to take for fibromyalgia because it rarely eases the pain and because aspirin aggravates irritable bowel syndrome, which is a common symptom of fibromyalgia. It turned out that a common symptom of fibromyalgia is a sudden weight gain due in part to the amount of fluid one retains in swollen joints and to the fact that mobility is restricted.

So did the first rheumatologist treat me poorly because I was fat? He treated poorly some of the other fibromyalgia sufferers who were *not* fat. Did he treat me poorly because he didn't believe in the existence of fibromyalgia? Did the association of fibromyalgia with weight gain and fatness color his judgment as to its legitimacy? Was he merely incompetent?

I really can't know for sure. But as I had in the case of the harassing staff member, I did know some important things.

I knew I hurt and that I didn't deserve to hurt. I knew I needed medical care. I knew this guy was not going to give me that care. I knew that I was going to have to find someone who would. I knew that whether he was well-motivated, had ulterior motives, or was just ignorant was irrelevant to my needs. His actions counted more than his intentions.

In the war on fat, it is impossible to tell which person is well-meaning, which person is simply lacking empathy, and which person is plainly out to get me. Bigotry works that way.

Most people do not think of themselves as practicing bigotry. Most people repeat something, perform some action, or ignore someone else's words or actions that are bigoted. Indeed, the battle I fight sometimes includes questioning my own thinking and my own feelings about fatness and fat people.

I prefer to model the enemy as a set of ideas that get repeated without examination within the culture. Some people profit greatly from this set of ideas and will support any effort to maintain these ideas as *truisms,* that is, as something so basic one should not take the time to examine closely. Some people mindlessly repeat these ideas, but when someone points out to them the problems with the ideas, they are willing to change their minds and sometimes their actions.

It takes practice to recognize bigotry and to challenge it in its many forms. It takes a strong mind willing to examine and reflect upon these truisms. It takes practice not to repeat these ideas and to recognize the repetition when it occurs.

Fighting ideas is difficult. It means that sometimes I have to confront friends and well-meaning strangers with the implications of what they are saying or doing.

It is easy to get angry with government officials, health researchers, street-level bureaucrats, and media moguls who pass along these ideas, because these people are not a part of my personal life. But the repetition of these ideas in everyday life is a necessary element to turn government policy, pseudo-scientific studies, and stereotypes into cultural givens.

I am a reluctant warrior. I did not choose this war, and I don't particularly like fighting the ideas that people have about fat people, about me.

I, like many other fat people, have politely listened to horrible things being said about my body or about bodies similar to mine, worried that saying something would mean someone would think less of me. I want to be liked. I want my skills and talents to be appreciated. I want my education to be of use to others. I want my life to be full and to be surrounded by people I love and who love me. In other words, I want pretty much what most people want. I want to be human.

But I have come to the conclusion that the only weapon I have as a fat person is to speak my mind. I have the advantage of living on the wrong side of many of the ideas that are repeated about fat people. That point of view has much to teach others.

I know that I risk ostracism, ridicule, and harassment for speaking out, but I also know that I am ostracized, ridiculed, and harassed even when I don't speak up.

The central fact that I have had to learn is that people will make up their minds about what my fatness means to them without my saying a single word. If they are afraid of fat, hate fat, or are just uncomfortable with fat, my body will bother them. My fear of not being liked is immaterial in the face of the fact that most people in this society probably already don't like me and are already offended by my body.

But just like the agents in *The Matrix,* the ideas that people have about fat are often not of their own making. They are repeating things to which they have given little or no thought. If they are truly my friends, my speaking to them about those enemy ideas has more of a chance of changing their minds than my remaining silent. Remaining silent weakens my mind and allows the negative ideas about my body and my life to take over my thinking.

Speaking my mind strengthens my mind, no matter what the immediate reaction from the listener. Speaking my mind has the possibility of changing someone else's mind and stopping the mindless repetition.

One central belief fuels the government policy makers, obesity researchers, street-level bureaucrats, and media: the social-problems claim that being fat is bad. Without this belief, the diet-pharmaceutical industrial complex and the accompanying social-problems industry would not carry on.

My enemy is this belief, and as a reluctant warrior I know that wherever this belief rears its ugly head, I must fight, even if I lose some friends along the way. I must speak my mind.

┌───┐
│ *Building Block #2:*   │
│   │
│   *Take your place.*   │
│   │
└───┘

I am continually amazed at the extent to which

I am expected to keep my mouth shut about things that pertain to my body. It is as if the anger of a fat person is the most dangerous thing in the world.

Asking for a chair without arms in places where I can find no place to sit is considered a radical act. I really don't know why it is considered a radical act, but from the reactions I receive, it is apparent that it is.

Most places will accommodate. Most are willing to do *something*. But often that something comes with a lecture about how nobody else has ever complained. Often that *something* comes with a smart aleck remark that isn't quite an insult, but stings nonetheless. Sometimes that *something* comes with an admonition that I should lose weight. Rarely, but occasionally, I've been told to go elsewhere, or that there is nothing they can do because even though *they* are sitting on a chair without arms, there are none available to the public. A couple of times I have been told that I would break their chairs and to get out. None of these *"somethings"* are pleasant.

Neither the medical system in the United States nor the one in Canada really cares about the health of fat people. I know this because the seating in doctors' offices and hospital waiting rooms is frequently too small for anyone weighing over 200 pounds. I cannot tell you the number of times I've sat in a waiting room crammed full of weight loss material with flyers on the wall encouraging people to inquire about various weight loss services, and none of the seats are wider than 16 inches, barely accommodating anyone with hips larger than 40 inches.

Exactly where would these fat people sit when they came to lose weight? Have these places found a miracle drug or procedure that ensures a patient will fit in those seats by their next visit?

A few years ago when my lupus and fibromyalgia were much worse and I was learning how to live with chronic illness, I found the professional conventions I attended a couple of times a year difficult.

Both lupus and fibromyalgia are autoimmune disorders. A stimulus that isn't particularly harmful to my body can potentially trigger an immune response that causes me pain. Sunshine is one of those stimuli. When I have been exposed to direct sunlight or halogen lighting for 20 minutes or more, I sometimes feel feverish and have flu-like symptoms with achy joints and a general feeling of uneasiness. This is not an uncommon experience among people with lupus.

Hotels where conventions are held are filled with large windows, skylights, and halogen lighting. So even if I stay indoors, I can develop a flare-up. As a consequence, in order to keep up and enjoy the convention, I usually bring a cane and wear sunscreen and a hat. Through medication and better care of myself, these flare-ups are rarer now, but I have to be cautious nonetheless.

I was at a convention a few years ago in a bright sunshiny city in the southern United States. By the second day of the four-day event, I was in pain and in need of my cane to get around. On the third night of the event, a banquet was held with a speaker I admired and whom I looked forward to seeing. Even though I was a graduate student and living on a strict budget at the time, I paid the $30 for the banquet.

It was held at a restaurant about five blocks from the main hotel. It was up a hill. I scouted all this out and left an hour early to ensure that I could take my time and rest along the way. It was a struggle, but I made it.

When I arrived at the restaurant, however, I discovered that a venue had been chosen in which the banquet facilities were upstairs with only a long, steep set of stairs to gain access. My choices were to forego the banquet and lose my $30 and miss the speaker, be carried up the stairs on a chair by four waiters, or walk the stairs. I opted for number three.

By the time I reached the top of the stairs I was in immense pain. My hips, knees, ankles, and toe joints were burning, and my legs felt like they were on fire. I made it to the restroom, where I broke down and wept, hoping that none of my colleagues could hear or identify me. This was a professional situation, and I felt ambushed, betrayed, and extremely vulnerable.

I recomposed myself. Then I got angry. On top of all the other struggles to get there, the banquet was overbooked and had too many people for the venue. While the chairs had no arms, they were pushed together tightly around long tables. We were rubbing against each other, so my burning legs were continually being re-stimulated, making relief from the stairs and hill impossible.

I smiled and chatted like nothing was going on, but the more I hurt, the angrier I got. As I looked around the room and saw women in their 70s and 80s who were also obviously struggling with the stairs and the crowded situation, the angrier I got. I also realized that like me, there might have been younger people who had struggled but didn't have the physical markings to suggest the internal pain.

I sat there in pain getting angrier and angrier, wondering why in a city this large, nine years after the passage of the Americans with Disabilities Act, someone would pick a crowded, inaccessible place to have a banquet.

Then I spotted one of the committee members who had been responsible for arranging the fiasco. I resolved that I was not going to make it through the evening. I had a long walk ahead of me back to the hotel. I was in too much pain to keep up the schmoozing for long. I was in no mood to listen to the topic of the evening or to meet the speaker I admired. The evening was ruined, and I just wanted to rub analgesic cream on my aching legs and try to get some sleep. So, having spotted the committee member, I resolved to say my piece and leave.

I sat down beside her and leaned over and asked a simple question: "Excuse me, but did the committee know that this restaurant was so inaccessible to disabled people when it was chosen?"

The woman looked at me as if I had called her a whore. "Well," she responded indignantly, "*we* can't think of everything."

Being nice was way beyond my ability at this point. I looked her straight in the eye and said, "This has been the worst experience I've ever had in this organization. It has been nine years since the law said a place like this should accommodate disabled people. You *should* have thought about this. You don't have an excuse." Then before she could respond, I got up and left.

I found this exchange especially enlightening because it occurred less than 24 hours after a dinner conversation with an African American woman who was complaining that the old guard of the organiza-

Yogurt

I sit in the kitchen, unable to sleep. My husband snores gently from the other room. I am adept at finding things in the dark so as not to wake my husband. Years of insomnia have trained me well.

Yogurt calms my stomach, sometimes. Smooth, creamy, fruity yogurt. I eat by the glow of the refrigerator light. Calmness fills the kitchen. Sometimes the middle of the night is my favorite time and space.

I close my eyes with each delicious bite. Suddenly, it is the summer of 1976.

"Have some, it's good." My roommate is sitting in our kitchen, also unable to sleep. It is 3 A.M.

I balk at first, crinkling my nose at a new experience. Unsure at first. Then, surrendering to the moment, I say "why not?"

I am won over by the smooth, creamy, cool taste on a hot Florida summer night. My first taste of yogurt.

1976 is a summer of firsts. It is the first time I have lived

tion was interested in encouraging African American participation, but wasn't interested in that participation actually changing anything. This is a common problem for organizations that give lip service to diversity without thinking through what encouraging that diversity means. It means that things have to change.

Organizations reflect the perspectives of their leaderships, including their cultural and social backgrounds. Organizations designed by white, upper middle class, well-educated and able-bodied baby boomers, even if those people happen to be women, will reflect the cultural and social values of white, upper middle class, well-educated, able-bodied people who were born around the same time. If those organizations become truly inclusive, they will undergo changes because the new people with different cultural and social backgrounds will bring their perspectives.

---

away from school and home, sharing an apartment. It is the first time I have learned to swim in the deep end of the pool. It is the first time I openly drink wine at parties and, at least, play like I am an adult.

It is the first time I try to be single at college. I broke up with my high school sweetheart before he left to go back home for the summer. He is the only boy I have ever kissed. I believe he is the only boy who has ever been interested in me. I am sure no one else will ever be interested again unless I lose 35 pounds. Looking back, I know this is not true, but at the time, it is what I believe.

A friend from my hometown sleeps in our living room because he doesn't like his un-airconditioned dorm room. My roommate and I laugh as he snores, unaware of our yogurt raid.

My friend has flirted with me a lot this summer, but I really don't understand the flirtation until years later. I am basically clueless most of the time. I am the "fat" girl, and no one would ever flirt with me.

"*WE* can't think of everything" is a red flag. If an organization systematically ensures that the leadership remains homogeneous in background and opinion, then no new thoughts will occur.

It is not necessary for an elite group of people to think of everything. If something is being left out, it is being left out because those people making decisions are excluding important points of view. I can assure you that if a disabled woman had been on that committee, she would have noticed the inaccessibility of the restaurant. *She* would

---

I work in the school mail room. It is hot and I wear shorts and a tank top to work most days. My supervisor has chased me around tables and left pornography open on my desk when his wife, who also works in the mail room, isn't around. It will be years later before I learn the words "sexual harassment."

The other student worker knows how uncomfortable I have been with the supervisor. He has offered to go to the administration and report the supervisor, but I don't want to make any trouble.

I voted for the first time this year. I voted for Jimmy Carter both in the primary and in November.

It is a wonderful time. It is a coming of age. It is a funky apartment with funky people and I should be enjoying every minute of it.

Isn't it funny how just the taste of yogurt can bring back so many memories?

But I didn't really experience any of these things when they happened. I feel them only in retrospect. I essentially missed the experience. The moment passes and I cannot get back the feeling again. The chance is gone. I was too busy worrying about my weight.

I had gained 25 pounds my freshman year at college, and I spent the first half of the summer starving myself, running or swimming every chance I got, trying to lose those unsightly pounds. I spent the month of August in bed, exhausted and

---

have thought of it.

Having lupus and fibromyalgia flare-ups is disabling at times. Being fat is not a disability. Being fat should be accommodated, however. Accommodating diversity is not about making everyone look or act the same way. We live with a number of accommodations in our everyday life.

Most cars have adjustable seats. Facial makeup comes in a variety of shades because skin color comes in a variety of shades. Almost

---

fighting a cold.

By the end of the summer, I weighed 35 pounds more than I did when I started college. But I could tread water.

By the end of summer, I reconciled with my high school sweetheart, decided he was the only person in the whole wide world who would ever love a fat girl like me so I had better do whatever it took to keep him, and got engaged.

By the end of summer, I decided that I had better play it safe.

By the end of summer, I had made my choices, and I still have to live with the consequences of those choices.

Yogurt in the middle of the night held such creamy promises of a sensual life. I look back and wish I had been more daring. Maybe I should have had the black cherry and chocolate instead of the strawberry.

I heard today a definition of "puritanical"—the fear that somebody, somewhere is having fun.

Maybe I should have invited my friend on the sofa to join us.

Maybe I should wake up my husband and have him join me the next time I eat yogurt in the middle of the night.

Hmmmmm.

every home has a stepladder because not everyone can reach into high cabinets or storage places. Bicycles come in 22-inch, 24-inch and 26-inch wheels with adjustable seats to accommodate different leg lengths. Shoe sizes vary. Language translators make good livings assisting in cross-cultural government or business interactions. These accommodations are made because human beings have a variety of physical characteristics, cultural backgrounds, tastes, talents, and skills.

Decisions not to accommodate difference are made on the basis of a belief that the difference is not worthy of accommodation. Some people have a preference for activities and objects that are harmful to other people. These preferences are not accommodated because they are deemed not worthy, and much of the time for good reason.

There are many things that can be put clearly in one category or the other with little debate or negotiation. However, there are also many things that cannot be as easily categorized. When confronting these gray areas, making accommodations for other characteristics, tastes, talents, and skills is negotiated in everyday interactions. These negotiations are made in the context of knowledge, skills, biases, prejudices, beliefs, and fears.

I have many critiques of health care in the United States, but there is one piece of health care legislation for which I have nothing but admiration: the Americans with Disabilities Act (ADA) passed in 1990. The law is simple in concept. It suggests that in order to ensure that business and organizational transactions are fair for people of differing abilities, a reasonable accommodation must be made.

The concept of "reasonable accommodation" is especially useful. The law outlines a *process* of finding reasonable accommodation, not an *outcome* regarding what that accommodation should be.

That process includes both the needs of the organization and the needs of the individual. It is the responsibility of the individual to make an organization aware of the particular needs, but once aware, the organization is responsible to negotiate an accommodation. Different kinds of negotiations are possible depending upon what kind of relationship is in question.

For example, an employer would not be expected to train a disabled person simply because they are disabled. But a qualified disabled person might reasonably expect to be hired even though hiring them may require modifications to the office environment in which they work.

A different example would be a business transaction between a customer and a business. Cruise ships are expected to provide accessible rooms with doors wide enough to accommodate wheelchairs. However, these modified rooms often cost more than the least expensive rooms on the ship. It is considered reasonable that the accommodations are available and that they are not the most expensive room on the ship. However, the law does not insist that such accommodations have to match the least expensive accommodations. Because the room has to be of a certain size in order to accommodate wheelchairs, pricing those rooms in the same range of equally sized rooms is a reasonable

Micro Insidiousness

I can't believe what just happened.

I'm sitting in Starbucks writing this book and across the room three children are laughing and pointing at me. I look straight at them and they look back and laugh.

"Mom, mom," they shout as they leave the building. "Did you see that fat woman?"

Mom is not only thin, she has an obvious boob job. She does not correct the children. She tells them to hurry along, as if I am poison or a monster.

As she gets out of earshot, I notice two Japanese businessmen in the corner looking at her as she leaves. They, too, are pointing, though more subtly than the children were. The smiles on their faces do not indicate ridicule and fear, but admiration and sexual attraction.

It is at these moments that I want to stand up and shout, "What is wrong with you people?"

In these small micro-interactions of people passing each other in the business of life lie the insidious mechanisms of stigma.

accommodation.

I like this law because it is flexible and it is practical. One does not have to worry about diagnoses or prognoses; one looks at functionality. It does not matter if a deformed leg or arthritis is the reason for a special chair, only that a special chair is needed. The emphasis is on the practical questions of space and mobility.

The thing I do not like about the ADA is that it is limited to questions of disability. It requires people to be divided into two categories: abled and disabled. The truth about abilities is that all people have varying needs.

Wouldn't it be a wonderful world where physical differences among people could be accommodated? The values upon which the Americans with Disabilities Act is based could provide a process for accommodating differences without having to put people in specific categories.

Fat activists have mixed feelings about the ADA. Fat people are often not disabled; however, the ADA offers their best chance of being accommodated in specific cases. It is a fine line to walk, and an extremely unfair position in which fat people find themselves.

Politically, using the ADA to negotiate accommodations means reinforcing a view of fat people as diseased. Personally, in order to make a living, to attend school, to engage in commerce or to sit in a public place, the ADA offers some fat people the best chance of getting something done.

In a fat neutral world, such a request for accommodations would be natural. Why wouldn't a place of commerce or education want to ensure that their clientele are comfortable?

But we do not live in a fat neutral world. In the current anti-fat climate, it is risky to raise the issue of accommodations. That is why I always laugh when someone says to me, "Well, no one else has mentioned that the seating is too small before." Such a statement is not much of a defense, and is mostly reflexive in nature.

However, I don't doubt its honesty. Look around sometime and ask yourself how many people look comfortable in their seats. I have seen fat people and short people and tall people looking extremely uncomfortable in a number of situations where seating is homogenous. Most people do not speak up. They remain uncomfortable and then wonder why they hurt at the end of the day.

My response to such a statement is, "Well, I'm telling you about it now."

My first clue that I am in hostile territory is that there are no chairs without arms.

Physical environments reflect social mores. Designing and decorating physical spaces are decisions that are made in a particular point in history, by specific people with specific goals in mind. This means that designing and decorating physical spaces reflect what is and is not important to the people making the decisions.

The absence of chairs that accommodate a variety of people is reflecting a design that does not consider diversity of bodies as important. It may be a sin of commission or omission, but it still means diversity was not a part of the social conscience of the designer(s).

Fat people are often accused of being lazy, inactive, or reclusive. Yet one of the reasons I often refrain from going out to restaurants, theatres, and other public places is that I am never going to be sure I will have a comfortable place to be when I get there.

Many people take for granted that where they go will be relaxing, offering an evening of entertainment. I do not take that for granted. I have to know if a new place will have an alternative for me. I have to know if setting up that alternative will be treated as a big deal or as natural.

There are places and activities I just avoid because I will be so weary from the machinations I have to go through just to have a place to sit. By the time the details have been worked out, I'm exhausted and unable to enjoy whatever it is that I came to see or experience.

The activity level of fat people is a chicken-and-egg question. Of course, it would be good for all people to be more physically active. Of course, movement is good for all of us. People derive great benefit from moving their bodies. People derive great benefit from being social. People derive great benefit from being part of a culture. But years of negotiation, stigmatization, and out-and-out hatred can push even the most outgoing of us indoors and in hiding. So how can we know if fat people are inactive because they are fat or because they are stigmatized?

We can't. I know that both sides have arguments, but in the current cultural environment we just can't know.

In larger cities and in specific cases there are fat friendly or size acceptance Meccas that offer safe spaces to be a large person. These places are used frequently, and one might argue this demonstrates that fat people would be more active in a fat neutral world. But one could easily argue that such places work only in urban areas because only a small percentage of fat people would be active, and only in urban areas are there enough such fat people to keep these organizations going.

Because the world is not fat neutral, we simply cannot know what would happen to fat people in a fat neutral world. But I would like to find out.

I would love to see a fat neutral world. I would like to see a world in which everyone was reasonably accommodated. That is the world for which I reluctantly fight. That is the place in which I'd like to be.

Historically, in Greek society, a stigma was a mark placed upon a person to denote a status. For example, a slave was given a stigma so he or she could not blend into the general population and pass for a free person. Over the years, the word came to have religious and psychological meanings, as some Catholics were said to spontaneously generate marks of religious symbolic meaning and some psychologists treated patients who believed they had spontaneously generated the same marks. Eventually, "stigma" came to mean any attribute or characteristic that makes a person seem less desirable or credible.

Goffman described stigma as a social process rather than an attribute. The process involves a particular physical or personal characteristic that is regarded as negative, the stereotypes about the particular characteristic that tell people to be leery of the stigmatized person, and the social circumstance that suggests what both the "normal" and the "stigmatized" person should do.

Some stigmas are visible, making the stigmatized person discredited upon first encounter. Other stigmas are invisible, making the stigmatized person discreditable, only having a spoiled identity, if the stigma is found out.

The elements of stigma, stereotypes, times and places of encounters, visibility of the stigma, and fears of being found out combine to create a number of possible outcomes with each social encounter.

For people with visible stigmas, such as a fat person, choices for managing the impressions other people have of them are limited. A fat person can overcompensate for fatness and try to make an impression that essentially cancels out the impression being fat makes. A fat person can withdraw and only interact with trusted friends and family. A fat person can become militant and remain in an adversarial position with others. A fat person can try to get thin.

Conventional beliefs suggest that weight loss is the only solution to the stigma of fat, but losing weight is an extremely difficult choice to pull off for any length of time. Besides that, there is always the question of how much thinner is enough. Going by the BMI standard, you could have a body like Brad Pitt or Lucy Lawless and still be considered fat. Going by popular culture, you could have a body like Ted Danson or Kate Winslet and still be considered fat.

My parents called me "Patsy" until second grade, when I found out my name was really "Patricia." I wanted to be known as "Pattie," and I chose the spelling to distinguish myself from all the other girls named "Patty." This turned out to be a disaster (in my seven-year-old mind) because, even though as a kid I was tall and skinny until I went through puberty, my schoolmates called me "Fatty Patty" or "Fat-Pat." When I started putting on some weight after puberty, I insisted on being known as "Tricia" to avoid the rhyme that in my mind was coming true.

The point is that fatness is a category that is ill-defined and is used to discredit people no matter what their body weight or fat-to-muscle ratio actually is. So losing weight might not work in removing the stigma even if it were possible to lose weight and keep it off. The truism "You can never be too rich or too thin" ensures that even the smallest among us can be discreditable as "too fat."

In his book *Our Kind of People,* about upper class African Americans, Lawrence Otis Graham wrote in his final chapter about passing for white, specifically the technologies employed in passing. Lighter-skinned African Americans often had plastic surgery to enhance their whiter characteristics.

But technology was not enough. In order to succeed at "passing," a person would have to cut off all ties with relatives and friends. He or she would have to watch his or her speech patterns and mannerisms constantly. She or he would usually not have children for fear that the child's features would betray their African heritage. It was a lonely and fearful existence for most.

The closet experience of homosexuals might be an even better parallel to weight. Both groups are part of a larger community of people who do not share their biological makeup. Both groups have been medicalized strictly on the basis of belonging to their respective

Maybes

For weeks I watched his beautiful pale blue

eyes turn yellow and clouded. The strong, hardworking father I had known for 42 years was gone and a weak, yellowing, wasting body was left in his wake. Death of the liver is not a pretty way to leave this world.

I had come home from a conference several weeks earlier to a phone message that was garbled so badly I barely knew it was my father's voice. I called his house and got the same babbling. Something was wrong.

I called my parents' neighbor.

"You'd better come over here. Your mom is in the hospital with pneumonia and Ray seems very confused."

When I arrived, he seemed drugged or drunk. I wasn't sure what was going on. He was not a drinker and was not on any medicine about which I knew. My husband and I stayed the night and in the morning he was better, but clearly something was wrong.

By the time mom was released from the hospital, dad was

groups. Both groups have a great deal of pressure to conform to what is an incredibly difficult standard for them to meet.

Of course, it is much harder to closet fatness than sexual orientation, but one might argue that weight loss for the larger person is a form of putting fat in the closet.

I have often wondered if losing weight is a means of "passing." My own experience is that I felt like I was passing for thin whenever I lost weight.

The most "successful" weight loss experience I had was when I lost 130 pounds in 18 months through the use of a synthetic amphetamine and, eventually, alcohol and Valium. To obtain and maintain this weight loss, I ate a thousand calories less a day than the WHO

---

not able to drive and didn't know where he was most of the time. We took him to his doctor.

"You've known about his liver condition for some time."

"Yeah, but he was getting better."

"The liver doesn't get better. Once it's damaged it's just a matter of time."

"What about transplants?"

"It's too far gone. He's not a good candidate for a transplant."

"Aren't there any medicines?"

"No. There's nothing we can do. I'm calling hospice and setting up a 'Do Not Resuscitate' order."

"Why didn't we see this coming?"

"It works like a step rotting from underneath. Everything looks fine until one day you step on the board and it falls apart underfoot. His liver just quit functioning."

"Will he be in pain?"

"No, he will slowly become more disoriented and unaware

---

standard for starvation. I walked and eventually ran two to four miles a day. When these drastic measures stopped working, I took Metamucil and Ex-Lax two to three times a week to "help out." I also frequently took a diuretic.

I got a physician to prescribe a diuretic for me because one time my blood pressure was measured as "high" and because my father had high blood pressure, establishing a "family history" excuse. The truth was that during the majority of my life, even when weighing over 200 pounds, my blood pressure stayed at normal to low range, and that my mother's family has *low* blood pressure. I often doubled the dose of the diuretic if I gained or hadn't lost weight in a particular week.

With all of this effort, I never got below 128 pounds. All my efforts and I still couldn't reach the supposed ideal 105 pounds for my five-foot-one-inch body. I was still "fat" according to the charts.

of his surroundings. He will most likely die quietly in his sleep."

He didn't steadily get worse. He got better for a few weeks. We had time for good-byes and thank-yous. We had time for what-ifs. While we waited and watched, it seemed like an eternity as he withered away before us.

Our days were filled with making him comfortable and taking care of his physical needs. For the last two weeks of his life, he was no longer recognizable. But the doctor was right, he was not in pain. When he finally passed, it seemed too short a time.

Attending the death of another being, especially a loved one, is a bittersweet experience. My dad was at his father's side when he passed. He had told me on several occasions how happy he was that he had been able to be there. He told me about the wonderment of watching all of the anguish of the stroke my grandfather had suffered leave his face with his last breath.

Being at my father's side felt like I had continued something important. I didn't understand exactly what, but I knew

I did none of these techniques openly. I knew that others would judge my behavior as unhealthy. And I knew that if I *appeared* alert and thinner, others would judge me as healthy and beautiful.

The craziness didn't stop at the secretiveness of the situation. I never felt comfortable. I felt like fat was going to break out at any moment.

I kept pictures of my fattest body not only to remind me never to get fat again and to keep motivated to continue these incredibly harsh and time-consuming measures, but also as proof that I was somebody else. If someone accused me of being fat, I could whip out the picture and say, "not any more."

My "before" picture proved my "after" existence because I was never comfortable with my "after" existence. I was ever vigilant.

My adult life can be divided into three distinct periods, with only

---

it was good. I felt his pulse slow and then stop. I heard his last breath. I cried. I still cry.

About a year after his passing, for some reason or another, I remembered a conversation I had with my father before he was diagnosed with liver damage.

"How are you feeling, Dad?"

"I'm having trouble breathing. I keep gaining weight. But I'm not eating anything except a little bit of apple sauce or oatmeal in the morning."

"Have you been to the doctor?"

"Yeah, he says I need to lose weight. But nothing I do seems to work. I don't know how to lose weight if I'm not eating anything."

"Did you tell him you weren't eating anything?"

"He doesn't believe me."

A month later my father was taken to the emergency room and 27 pounds of fluid was drawn from his abdomen. That was when they found out that his liver was damaged. They told

a few people privy to all three periods.

Until I lost the 130 pounds, I was fat and always trying to lose weight. There were other successful attempts, the second highest being the 85 pounds I lost on a liquid diet. But I never was "really" thin. After the age of 18 until I became addicted to diet pills and Valium, I never got below a size 16. No matter how much weight I managed to lose, I always considered myself a failure because I never reached the goal weight.

Then I lost half my body weight and got a divorce. When I left my first husband, I also left the majority of my friends. I truly started over. At my lowest point, I could wear a size 8. I didn't reach my goal of 115 pounds, which *still* would have been higher than the charts said

---

him he had six months to live. He lived 18 more months.

Hemochromatosis is a congenital condition in which a person does not process iron in the blood system correctly and it builds up in the liver, causing damage if left unchecked. My mom doesn't remember if the doctor diagnosed the hemochromatosis before or after Dad's visit to the emergency room.

To ensure that someone with hemochromatosis doesn't get liver damage, the patient has a pint of blood drawn weekly until he or she becomes anemic. The patient is not supposed to eat iron-enriched foods and has his or her blood monitored frequently. The test for iron in the blood is inexpensive and fairly easy to do. But there are no symptoms until there is damage, so the doctor has to be sensitive to family history. Blood iron levels are a regular screening.

My father did not go to doctors until late in life. He did not have regular screenings, and therefore his condition went years without diagnosis.

Certainly, this delay contributed to his early death. By the time all the symptoms were sorted out the damage was done, and as the doctor said, the rotting had begun and it was just a

---

I should have been.

My work colleagues and new friends knew me as a "normal-sized" person. I'd shown some of them the pictures just to make sure they understood my bravery and struggle and success, but for the most part, I am certain these people pictured me as a petite, slightly plump runner. Some of them knew me as I started gaining the weight back, but as I gained weight, I became less social.

Then I decided to go back to school and lost touch with most of those folks. In school, I was a fat chick again, but I was becoming a lot more adamant about accepting my fatness.

These three identities had three distinct stories I told about my body. *Fat but trying to lose weight* told a story of unwanted fat. I was a

matter of time before the step fell through.

But I cannot get that conversation out of my head.

Did the doctor ignore the fluid retention so long that the damage was done? What if this were a fat neutral world where fat people aren't regarded as liars when they say they're not eating that much? Certainly, my father's sudden weight gain was a symptom that was ignored.

Maybe, in a fat neutral world, changes in weight would be regarded as symptoms rather than indictments.

Maybe all the money that was spent on figuring out how to make people lose weight could have been used to figure out how to repair damaged livers.

Maybe if the doctor had paid attention, he would have tested the liver three or four months earlier and started the blood-letting sooner.

Maybe my dad would have seen me graduate with a Ph.D. I am the first doctor of my generation on his side of the family.

Maybe instead of clouds gathering in his beautiful blue eyes, I would have seen pride.

Maybe.

thin person trying to break free of a fat body. *Thin, but fearful of gaining* told a story of tentative success and a fear of being found out as an inner fatty. I was a thin person on the outside, but I knew I could not maintain the incredible and increasingly failing methodology it was taking to pass for thin. *Fat but comfortable in my own skin* tells the story of struggle to be okay with myself in a world that would rather I not.

This third identity carries with it a sense of authenticity. I rarely feel like I'm inadequate or faking. Of course, I carry insecurity about all this, but I'm increasingly comfortable in my own skin, and I believe that comfort comes from living more authentically. By "authentic," I mean that my thoughts, beliefs, emotions, and outer body are more in sync with each other. I no longer feel at war with myself. I have taken my place in my world.

While I know that my experience with dieting and losing weight matches what I have read of the experiences of both visible minorities and homosexuals "passing," I also know that I cannot say all weight loss attempts are a form of passing. However, I would assert that the case for weight loss as a form of passing can be made, and that if we began to think of weight loss techniques as technologies for passing, it would change our view of them.

"Passing" implies a perceived superiority of the identity that we are trying to assume. It would benefit all of us if we were to reject the slender body as the only ideal, and embrace bodies of all sizes.

Passing, however, is an extreme example of something most of us do every day. Everyone attempts to manage the impression they make on others in everyday interactions.

We wear particular hairstyles, wear particular clothes, say particular things, avoid saying other particular things, drive particular cars, live in particular places and reveal particular personal biographical information, in part, to make an impression on the people around us. This is true even if the impression we are conveying is "I don't care about conventions."

For the most part, we do this without much thought. We know that when we go to an office setting we wear certain clothes, when we go to a wedding we wear certain clothes, and when we attend a sports event we wear certain clothes. We learned this at one point in our lives, but we do not always review the lessons later. We *just know.*

When any of us meets a stranger, we rely upon symbols such as clothing to tell us whether to welcome the stranger or to be leery of the stranger. These symbols are based upon things we have learned either from personal experience or from being taught by others. Some of these symbols make sense and are important in allowing us to anticipate social circumstances. If we did not have something upon which to rely to anticipate social situations, we would constantly be reinventing the social wheel, so to speak, having to relearn things on a daily basis. Thus, having these symbols enhances social circumstances and increases the possibility of building social relationships that we need.

Some of these symbols are based on stereotypes that serve to cut off potential relationships rather than enhance social circumstances. Goffman understood stigma to be a process of managing a spoiled image (stigmatization) in the presence of stereotypes about that image. "Passing" as a method of managing one's image relies upon the stereotypes remaining in place, because they help keep the secret identity secret.

In the war on fat, a fat warrior's battleground is not the stigmatized characteristic (fatness), but the stereotypes that have been built up through standards of beauty, economic interests, political alliances, and mindless repetition of what has become taken for granted about fatness.

One approach to this war would be to rely upon what I consider to be the obvious point, that society pays a price for excluding certain people just on the basis of how they look. Many fat people are talented, skillful, joyful, and interesting people whose potential contributions to the world around them are being lost due to the stigma placed on them. I want to shout, "Isn't it obvious that such prejudice will just hurt everyone?" But drawing a line in the sand and declaring something to be "just wrong" is usually not an effective strategy for changing culture.

Culture is built largely on repetition of words, images, and thoughts. The battleground of the war on fat is wherever the idea that "fat is bad" (or its equivalents, such as "fat is ugly," "fat is dirty," "fat is ignorant," "fat is unwanted," fat is unsightly," "fat is lazy," "fat is unhealthy," and so forth) is repeated.

A reasonable argument will not make an idea go away. It helps those who are willing and ready to stop and think about fatness, but most people do not stop and think about most of the *givens* that they hold. "Fat is bad" is an extremely embedded *given* in this society. If we are to eradicate this idea, we will have to repeat other messages, loudly and often. Stereotypes are most often *replaced* rather than erased.

Stereotypes have histories usually connected to colonization. When an imperialistic culture conquers another culture, they historically have imposed their culture on the conquered. This is done for several reasons.

First, to govern, the conquerors must ensure communication takes place efficiently. Forcing the conquerors' language onto the conquered helps ensure that.

Second, to act imperialistically, the conquerors usually share a belief in the superiority of their culture over others. This assertion of the newly dominant culture as uniformly superior leads to a necessary disrespect for the conquered culture. To survive under the new rule, many of the conquered people will adapt and learn the conqueror's culture.

Third, even if the conquerors do not believe in their own superiority, the strategy of controlling cultural exchanges is a good strategy to keep populations under control. There is a reason that totalitarian or invading regimes take control of art, music and media production. Controlling culture is a way of controlling minds.

Finally, as part of the imperialistic campaign, breaking up the conquered culture is a good strategy to enable the conquerors to impose their will. Stereotypes about the conquered people grow out of this strategy. These stereotypes usually involve beliefs that the conquered people are lazy, dirty, ignorant, and undesirable (except as potential exotic objects or fetishes).

In the past 60 years or so, a number of formally conquered peoples have gained independence or at least some semblance of independence from their colonizers. Part of the process of fighting off the stereotypes placed upon them has been to reclaim their former culture. Sometimes this is impossible because so much has been lost, but having a history creates a sense of community and commonality upon which a group of people can build something distinct and human—in other words, something that replaces the stereotypes.

The civil rights movement was not merely a legal battle. It involved reclaiming African symbols and incorporating slave narratives into freedom stories in order to teach those with such a heritage that they have value, meaning, and connection to their cultural past.

Aboriginal peoples around the world have used a reconnection to their language, religion, and culture to strengthen their bonds and differentiate themselves from the stereotypes that dominant cultures have about them. Neighborhoods of immigrants, reserves and reservations, and just the ease by which people who share common languages and histories can group together, allow for organized efforts to challenge stereotypes and dominant cultural beliefs, replacing them with old traditions and newly acquired self images.

Other groups like feminists and homosexuals have found commonality in experience.

Second-wave feminism built its movement on more than challenging gender discrimination. Middle and upper class white women were historically put in domestic situations where contact with the outside world was limited. After experiencing some independence in munitions factories during World War II, in the post-war U.S. many of these women moved with their husbands to the newly invented suburbs. With their houses closer together, women began to have more frequent contact with each other.

At first, the discussion topics were domestic in nature. However, proximity allowed for consciousness-raising groups to emerge. Some women began to see the commonality of their experiences and began to critique the stereotypes that kept them from public domains. They began to replace feminine stereotypes with powerful images of working women who could "bring home the bacon and fry it up in a pan."

Homosexuals, by virtue of needing places where they could meet and find loving relationships, and by virtue of the fact that their loving relationships were being stigmatized, created an underground of meeting places. In the 1950s, these were centers of creative activity and, in contrast to the emerging suburban landscape, some of these poets, songwriters, and performers were coming out of the closet with little consequence.

But by the 1960s, a backlash against gay culture occurred in the United States. Homosexuality and the underground hangouts of homosexuals were made illegal. A renewed interest in calling homosexuality a disease led to an increase of specialists and treatment programs aimed at cures.

However, the more homosexuality was criminalized, medicalized, and harassed, the stronger the cultural bond of homosexuals became. The explosion of anger and force marking the milestone protest and riots at the police raid of Greenwich Village's gay Stonewall Inn in 1969 was built upon the necessity of creating cultural connections in order to survive.

The politics of the gay rights movement were born out of these cultural connections. Stereotypes of gay men and lesbian women have been replaced with images of strong human beings who take pride in who they are and celebrate their differences.

Stereotypes regarding dark-skinned people, people who do not speak English, women, and homosexuals do still circulate in the culture. However, by the 1980s it was considered so impolite or unethical to mention these stereotypes in public that the term "political correctness" arose to describe the social expectation not to evoke such stereotypes in conversation even if one still believed the stereotype to be true.

Many complain of not being able to speak their prejudices. Others fear that something they say or do may be regarded as prejudice. Even with such tensions, many people have had a change of heart because the cultural landscape has changed.

Replacing stereotypes about fat is going to be more difficult.

Fat people have remained isolated from each other for the most part. There is no common cultural history or language to be reclaimed, because fat people come from all ethnic backgrounds and speak many languages. There is no ghetto, neighborhood, or common meeting place (except weight loss groups, where only those losing weight may speak) that facilitates group cohesion. There are few fat underground meeting places for fat people to find partners, because many fat people are as affected by the standards of what is an attractive mate as are thinner people, and don't always look for other fat people as mates.

There have been attempts at creating such meeting places. The Fat Underground was formed in the early 1970s because of the realization that feminists were not questioning the imperative to be thin and the National Association for the Advancement of Fat Acceptance (NAAFA) was not questioning patriarchy. The valiant efforts of the Fat Underground are still influential in the war on fat, but the Fat Underground has not grown into an extensive underground in the same way that bathhouses, bars, bookstores, and cafes have become "gay" hangouts.

A number of medical, legal, and economic arguments have been raised in an effort to end the war on fat. Some health professionals have challenged obesity research on scientific grounds. Fat people in the U.S. have come together to challenge discrimination practices in the law in efforts that have included anti-discrimination laws being enacted in four cities and one state. Fat-owned and fat-accommodating businesses have sprung up, and some marketing reports have suggested catering to larger clients is the new hot market.

I am appreciative of these actions and arguments, which help most because they offer new ideas to replicate within a culture. Certainly medical, legal and economic authorities originate many of the ideas we repeat, even if we do not hear them directly from those authorities. But, sadly, I do not believe this will be enough to win the war. These changes cannot simply be made on the margins of society, and they cannot be made in top-down efforts originating from a small group of experts.

Fat people are not a minority. Currently the American government defines 65 percent of its population as being fat.

A number of fat activists have asked why, more than 30 years after the formation of the Fat Underground, we still do not have a viable and powerful fat political movement.

The answer is that fat people have no culture to which they can return. The answer is that fat people have no ghetto or suburb where they can meet. The answer is that fat people do not seek out only other fat people in order to form loving relationships or to create a family unit. The answer is that being fat does not automatically create commonality, except through the cultural stereotype. The answer is that most fat people suffer the consequences of being stigmatized in silent solitude, internalizing a hatred for themselves and conspiring with their culture to keep up the stereotypes about who they are. The answer is that unlike other stigmatized groups, the way out of this big fat mess is through the center.

Fat hatred is so completely marbled into the dominant culture that only a radical change to the culture will shake the war on fat.

Fat hatred is steeped in the common fear that all people have about their acceptability to others. Fat hatred is steeped in the alienation that has been cultivated in order to sell solutions in a culture that looks to consumption as salvation.

Fat hatred is a culture hating what it sees in the mirror and then ostracizing the ones among us who remind us of that hatred most.

Fat hatred is evident in the medicalization of fat by the creation of a medical condition called "obesity."

Under the dominant paradigm of Western medicine,[7] diseases have causes and effects. Such an understanding of health is challenged when risk factors cannot account easily for incidences of disease. Many researchers cling to the rhetoric of the dominant paradigm in part because examining the complicated relationship between body size, lifestyle choices, and health shakes up the whole risk factor model of health.

Researchers want to be able to quantify physical phenomena, because it makes replication of studies possible and thus reliability easier to establish. Insurance providers want neat lists of diseases that are covered or not covered according to the diagnostic codes. Physicians want to be able to know when they have cured a patient and want to be able to avoid accountability when something goes wrong.

A nice linear model of risk factors and health makes the jobs of health professionals a lot simpler and easier. But a nice linear model is not always the most useful model of the relationship between risk factors and health.

Risk factors often imply cause and effect where such a relationship cannot be demonstrated. Three things are needed to demonstrate cause and effect:

1. There must be a correlation between the proposed cause and the proposed effect in which a change in the cause produces a fairly consistent change in the effect.

2. The proposed cause must occur in time before the proposed effect. This seems simple enough, but often it is difficult to prove.

3. No other explanation for the correlation can be found. That means that to be sure the argument made is valid, some thought and study must be given to the possibility of other explanations for the correlation that is observed. Among these other explanations is the possibility that these two factors are being caused by a third factor not being considered, or the two factors may have a relationship that looks strong when a third factor is present, but if one considers incidences when the third factor is not present, the relationship changes.

Even though the social-problems claim regarding the health crisis of obesity uses the language of cause and effect, most studies fail to consider the time sequence question or alternative explanations. For example, many studies do not study when or how a person gains weight and/or when or how a person develops a disease. The study merely notes that there is a higher prevalence of a certain disease among the fatter subjects than the thinner subjects.

If the fatter subjects became fatter *after* contracting the disease in question, it would be quite difficult to assert cause and effect in which weight causes the disease. The relationship could be reversed, with weight gain being a *symptom* of the disease.

Complicating this is the fact that a diagnosis may come much later than onset of a disease. So the question of when something happens often cannot even be answered, making it virtually impossible to assert a cause and effect relationship.

Wasted Words –

so much wasted words
calling small revolutions
of powerful shift-

key rhetoric: now
too much beauty is ignored
my life is too short-

shifted gears and stopped
playing the radio loud
turn all the way off

outside I hear
stiller's jays and dark ravens
keeping a beat in-

time with woodpeckers
drumming for their morning meals
caw, thump, coo, thump, trill

maybe love letters
will change more than protest songs
complaint letters fall

on deaf ears, cold hearts
love letters don't fall at all
but rather wiggle-

in and warm the heart
making room for making love
to a person's soul

Pattie Thomas
2003

Most of these obesity-related studies fail on the third account as well. These studies often are not designed to account for factors such as yo-yo dieting, level of activity, genetic makeup, or complicating lifestyle factors such as smoking, consumption of alcohol, or poor dietary habits.

They assume, but do not actually determine, that being fat reflects low levels of activity and poor dietary habits. Often size is used as a marker of lifestyle rather than studied as a separate factor. This leads to assertions such as the claim that there are 300,000 "obesity-related" deaths per year.

The research the "300,000 obesity-related deaths" assertion is based upon studied activity levels, diet, and mortality, not weight. The researchers spuriously generalized their findings to fat people, claiming increased mortality was related to obesity rather than to inactivity and nutrition, because everybody *just knows* fat people aren't active and eat poorly. There are other fallacies in the social claim besides the cause and effect problems.

Another problem with the linear model of risk and health is that proof of a correlation or even a causal relationship does not automatically suggest a solution.

There are a number of diseases that are correlated with particular characteristics of bodies. Because of the complex nature of genetics, physical characteristics often cluster together in regular patterns. Sometimes this is a matter of family lineage, with specific genetic characteristics being passed along with DNA. Sometimes it is environmental, in that people with certain physical characteristics have their life chances limited by the social stigma placed upon them through stereotypes and popular beliefs. In either case, one would be hard pressed to suggest that such a correlation could be changed by simply changing the body shape or physical characteristics.

"Passing" does not improve health. There is some evidence that being fat is mostly due to genetics. There is also some evidence that dieting and other forms of weight loss technologies cause harm. So even if there is a correlation between health and fatness, the next logical step is not necessarily weight loss. Prescribing weight loss might be the equivalent of prescribing skin lightener to cure sickle cell anemia. It might change appearances, but the inner biology remains.

Proof of a positive relationship does not prove a negative relationship. Even if we concede that being fat is correlated with or even causes certain diseases, few studies have been done to demonstrate that weight loss itself decreases these risks. One of the reasons few studies have been done is that it is very difficult to find enough people with significant weight loss for a long enough period of time to study the health benefits.

Sure, thinner people may have fewer incidences of certain diseases, but examining a cross-section of a population does not demonstrate that if individuals on the high end of the spectrum lose weight they will then experience the health benefits of those on the low end of the spectrum.

Finally, the relationship between being fat and being healthy is much more complex than a simple correlation suggests. A number of studies have suggested that there are *positive* relationships between health and fatness.

Works by Paul Ernsberger and Glenn Gaesser have outlined the benefits of body fat in fighting chronic and terminal diseases such as cancer and AIDS, and the potential protective benefits of fatness as suggested by lower incidence of several serious diseases in fat people. Fatness also interacts with ethnicity, family history, and genetic factors to paint an intricate and complicated picture—certainly, a picture nowhere near as simple as the diet-pharmaceutical complex would have us believe.

The battle of fat hatred is being fought every time a health expert reduces health down to risk factors. The complexities of the relationships between risk factors and disease undermine the view of the human body through the lens of size alone.

Fat hatred is grounded in a simplistic and reductionistic view of health that judges health by a single indicator, that is, weight. A holistic view of the human body has to allow for variations among those bodies. The battle of fat hatred is fought every time someone writes down a weight on a chart as an indicator of health.

The battle of fat hatred is being fought every time any of us looks in a mirror and worries about how acceptable her or his body is to others. One of the most telling examples of this is the coupling of "obesity" with eating disorders. How exactly do we tell young girls who are starving and purging in order not to get fat that being fat is another disorder? Doesn't defining fatness as a disease justify their efforts to get or stay thin? How narrow is the range of orthodoxy to be?

The doublespeak that occurs in such rhetoric is mind-boggling when examined closely. Paul Campos, in his book *The Obesity Myth*, quotes one young woman (who described herself as five-foot-seven and "107.3 pounds") stating, "I can't stand the idea of being fat. Even the word disgusts me. Overweight people want the world to accept them the way they are, so why can't people accept me the way I am?"

If fatness is an undesirable disease, her fat hatred and drastic means of staying thin make perfect sense.

The battle of fat hatred is fought every time we watch an advertisement and go shopping. Post-industrial capitalism is based upon advertisers convincing audiences they are in need of products. It is important that these products not fully satisfy the customer, because repeat business is the key to economic expansion.

Thus, the diet product is a perfect consumption product. It works just enough to convince the customer that it has potential, but not enough to succeed at permanent change. In fact, the customer is now convinced that any problems with the product are due to defects in the customer and not the product.

Can you imagine how your bargaining position would change in acquiring a new vehicle if every time it broke down, you felt guilty because the breakdown is taken as a sign of you being a bad owner? The price of cars would skyrocket, while the quality of the various models would probably never improve again.

The battle of fat hatred is fought every time a kid is bullied, harassed or admonished for how she or he looks. Fat is a prominent dynamic in the effort to make all of us under the control of a dominant paradigm that says we are not enough. This paradigm starts seeping into our consciousness and habits at early ages.

Every time a kid yells, "Look, mommy, that woman is fat," and is hushed up and rushed out of view, the kid learns "Fat is bad." The kid also learns the more general lesson that *difference* is bad. This ensures that telling a kid she or he is different can control her or his behavior for fear she or he will be considered bad as well. *Shut up. Don't look. Don't be one of them.*

No wonder kids bully. Things are set up so that bullying works very well.

The current lack of understanding of what fat is, how one gets fat, and whether one should want to be fat is an understanding that sets up a fear of fat. We are taught that on the thin to fat continuum, any particular person could end up running the gamut.

Many believe that everyone can be thin and everyone can be fat. Thin people are told that they are in constant danger of gaining weight and that a 10-pound gain could just as easily be a 100-pound gain. Fat people are told that they must lose weight and that a 100-pound loss is better than a 10-pound loss.

The truth is that many people, no matter how poor their eating and exercise habits, will remain thinner than average. The truth is that many people, no matter how healthy their eating and exercise habits, will remain fatter than average.

The belief that fat is bad, coupled with the belief that anyone could be fat if they were not careful, fuels fat hatred and keeps virtually everyone in the grip of the diet-pharmaceutical industrial complex. To change this paradigm, fat warriors must successfully challenge three cultural ideas.

First, they must challenge the basic idea that fat is bad. There are a number of ways this can happen within culture. One of the more positive ways to challenge this idea is for fat people to talk, write, and produce works of art reflective of their bodies and their experiences in their bodies.

The documentary *Fat Chance* follows the trials and tribulations of a 400-pound Manitoba man who attempts to lose weight and then decides to accept himself as he is. In the film, Rick Zakowich, the subject of the documentary, meets Lynn McAfee, one of the founders of the

Fat Underground, at a weekend retreat sponsored by the Association for the Health Enrichment of Large People (AHELP). McAfee tells Zakowich that she kept nothing but "fat art" in her home, stating that she was learning a "fat aesthetic." Culture is created by repetition and representation of values. For valuing fat and for fat people to become a part of the dominant culture, we must repeat and represent fatness as an acceptable aesthetic and a common experience.

Second, we must challenge the fear that anyone can be fat. Fatness is not a disease that anyone can catch. Fatness is not a condition that results from poor lifestyle. Fatness is not a moral question. "Fat" is merely an adjective describing the size of a body. This means that the concept of "obesity" must be challenged.

"Obesity" is a medicalization of fatness. It has no true basis in science. It might be reflective of a certain correlation between being fat and other diseases, but medicalizing that correlation is at best akin to suggesting that being African American causes sickle cell anemia, that being female causes ovarian cancer, and that being male causes male-pattern baldness.

The strongest defense against the fear of fatness has come from a growing number of researchers, health care workers, academics and other professionals who ascribe to the Health at Every Size (HAES) paradigm. HAES is based on the belief that weight or size has little to do with health, and that making it such an important indicator of health is actually hurting the medical treatment of all people.

Fat people often have a long list of doctor/patient stories in which they go to their doctor for treatment of a particular ailment and are told that whatever is wrong with them will not be cured until they lose weight. This list includes things like infections and diseases that have absolutely no established correlation to body size. On the other hand, thin people with serious health conditions that have a positive correlation to fatness often suffer from fat stigma as well, as doctors put off tests for diabetes or heart disease because the patient doesn't have the body type they associate with such diseases.

Symptoms misinterpreted through the doctor's cultural view of body size can spell disaster for a person of *any* size. Symptoms ignored by a doctor who justifies withholding medical care in order to induce a patient to lose weight can also be disastrous.

In addition, HAES proponents believe that all persons, no matter what size, can benefit from eating good food, eating when hungry, eating until satiation, and moving their bodies on a regular basis, *whether or not weight loss results.* A positive lifestyle is possible for anyone at any size, and size is not an indicator of that positive lifestyle.

A healthy weight is whatever weight a body is when it is receiving the nurturing and nourishment it needs. Weight is simply not that important an indicator, and should not be monitored or reviewed as an indicator.

Finally, we must challenge the economic forces that benefit from our dissatisfaction with our bodies. The current thinking among businesses is that people buy things because they want them, and the more they want something, the more willing they are to buy it. This belief about how value is created is relatively new. Historically and cross-culturally, there are other beliefs about why, when people exchange money, goods and services, they value items differently.

A growing number of people have begun to question consumption and the value system of satisfying wants that supports over-consumption. Unfortunately, many of those people have decided to use fat bodies as a symbol of over-consumption. This is sad, because fat hatred itself could be a symbol of the convoluted ways in which over-consumption is wasteful and harmful to human beings and other living things.

Diet products are wasteful because they are basically food, drugs, and supplements that are repackaged and sold at higher prices. On top of which, they do not achieve their explicit goal. The consumers of these products believe that the failure of these products is the consumers' own fault, so more money is spent on fruitless efforts. My guess is that unless I am alone in my experience with such products, many of them end up in landfills, half-used because they didn't work or people gave up on trying to make them work.

Health spas and gyms are able to stay in business not because they have a loyal clientele that comes to the facility regularly, but because most of their clientele only darken the doors of the facility upon occasion. Most of the larger gym chains stay in business because consumers who feel guilty about their bodies sign up for "mandatory" one or two-year minimum contracts and only come for a month or less. The money keeps pouring in, but no service or product has to be delivered. This is wasteful in time, effort, and exchange of funds.

Money that is used to fund the diet-pharmaceutical industrial complex's many pharmaceutical and medical procedures is also wasted. These resources and knowledge bases could be used for more productive and important matters such as universal health care, contagious disease control, and encouraging healthy lifestyle choices for ALL people.

Rejecting consumption as the basis for value would not mean wrecking the economy. An economy based on reasonable accommodation of all kinds of people would be a thriving economy, because it would put people first, and people have a variety of needs.

I am old enough to remember discussions of how in the 21st century, gadgetry and technology would allow human beings to pursue art, music, poetry, literature, and humanities with ease. We were supposed to have spare time to play and work. Instead, our so-called advanced civilization has created a system whereby most of us spend over 50 hours a week creating a "livelihood."

Supposedly, archeological evidence of past hunter/gatherer (so-called primitive) societies suggests that only 20 hours a week was spent by adults to provide food, shelter, and clothing for the members of their groups.[8]

Most contemporary American households require two adults to work full-time in order to meet the costs of running the house. There are people in the United States and Canada working two or three jobs and still living below the poverty level.

Fat hatred is part of a system of consumption that ensures escalating wastefulness because perpetual increase of the "needs" constructed by society ensures we will remain dissatisfied with ourselves. We are told that buying certain products will bring satisfaction, but even if it does so in the short term, the bar is always raised eventually to force additional consumption.

Fat people who do not try to lose weight are indeed a danger to that system. We are not terrorists. We are not costing the system too much. Rather, we stand as a symbol that it is possible to be satisfied with who we are right now, without having to purchase something in order to be somebody we are not.

This does not mean that we are refusing to participate in the exchange of goods and services. We consume, but that consumption is based on the value of who we are, not who we think or are told we should be.

The simple act of not spending money on the diet-pharmaceutical industrial complex seems like a radical act indeed. But in truth, it is an extremely ordinary act. We are satisfied with who we are. We ask only for the accommodations that should be afforded all human beings.

We intend only to take our place.

Building Block #3:

Follow your inner Sumo.

There are a number of names under which people fight fat hatred. Some people prefer "size acceptance" because it allows for an array of interests to be brought together in coalition. Businesses that cater to larger people are often said to be serving "the plus-sized market." This is a functional term, implying the meeting of needs without regard to why these people are larger or if they are trying to lose weight. "Health at Every Size" (HAES) was coined as a way of suggesting that concentrating on weight as a major health indicator hurts people of all sizes, not just fat people.

There are people who want to lose weight or are selling weight loss solutions who consider themselves to be fighting fat hatred as well. In the months I have been writing this book, I have mentioned the topic to a number of people, including friends, colleagues, and strangers. It is a rare moment when someone says to me something negative about it. The most negative reactions I have received have been that while the person was in agreement that fat people are stigmatized, she hoped I would not forget the health problems being fat "caused" (her exact word), and that I could help fat people with "their problem." Most people have told me they are sick of hearing about how North Americans are fatter, and they don't like the current bombardment of messages they are receiving everywhere they look.

Of course, I don't talk about the book or my feelings about fat with most people. I especially don't talk about the book, or my feelings, with people who harass me, who look at me funny, or who whisper and run away when they see me. So my sample, if one were to call it that, is highly biased.

Some people understand fat stigma and sympathize with the prejudice fat people face, and *still* believe that fat is bad or, at least, unhealthy. I know this is possible personally because not too many years ago I was saying the same thing. "I don't want to be skinny. I just want to lose a few pounds so I can feel better. I won't use harsh methods this time. I will lose weight sensibly."

The good news is that I've discovered I can feel better without losing any weight at all. In fact, I can feel healthier without even *considering* weight.

I have weighed myself only once in the past three years. I have days I feel bloated and heavy. I have days I feel light and energetic. I don't think my weight has anything to do with those feelings.

I do think that a good night's sleep, regular exercise, drinking lots of water, and eating when I'm hungry and finishing when I'm full does have a lot to do with it. However, I also think that lupus flare-ups, fibromyalgia flare-ups, and asthma attacks have something to do with those fluctuations as well. While I have influence on those flare-ups, I do not have control, and I have had to learn to accept that as part of my life.

In a sense, I am both healthy and unhealthy. On one hand, I function fairly well in life these days, especially compared to several years ago and to the six months I fought pneumonia. At this writing, I went for over a year without a cold or flu, and was able to fight a summer cold without an asthma attack or weeks in bed with bronchitis. I can tolerate more sunshine that I used to be able to tolerate, and I have more energy.

On the other hand, I have three incurable diseases that will affect my well-being for the rest of my life. Lupus, in more severe flare-ups, can be life-threatening. Asthma also can be life-threatening if untreated. Can someone with chronic, incurable diseases be called healthy?

The question is unanswerable as it is posed. But posing questions as "either/or" is exactly what is wrong with the current view of health in North American thought. "Either/or" questions usually leave out significant points of view.

Radley Balko, policy analyst with Cato Institute and a columnist for FoxNews.com, and Kelly Brownell and Marion Nestle, two prominent obesity researchers, squared off with each other over an either/or question posed by *Time* in its June 7, 2004 special issue on obesity. The question was: "Are you Responsible for Your Own Weight?" Balko took the "pro" side and Brownell and Nestle took the "con" side.

The argument is laid out on one page, with the "pro" on the left and the "con" on the right. In the middle of the page, there is a cartoonish picture of two disembodied hands holding what looks like part of a Russian matryoshka (nesting doll). The bottom left hand is holding half of the larger doll and the right hand is pulling (almost plucking) the smaller doll from the larger bottom. This illustrates the cultural understanding of fat as "obesity." Disembodied helpers who are working hard on behalf of the infantilized fat person to ensure that the thinner version of that fat person can emerge miraculously (after all, these hands look like the hands of God) from the fatter self.

The thinner doll is passive, looking downward, and seems to be making no effort whatsoever to assist in this transformation. This picture really *is* worth a thousand words about how the medical research establishment sees the fat body.

Below the headline exclaiming the question are sub-headings for each column, summarizing the position. Balko's "pro" is entitled: "Absolutely. Government has no business interfering with what you eat." Brownell and Nestle's "con" is entitled: "Not if blaming the victim is just an excuse to let industry off the hook."

It is interesting that Balko can speak in absolutes, putting the responsibility of fatness (and fat stigma) on the stigmatized other. The con side, however, is not defending fat people, per se. They still need changing. Instead, Brownell and Nestle try to remove scrutiny of their *own* industry ("obesity" research and "treatment") by placing blame on the food industry.

It's a debate about food, not fatness. Fatness, however, is assumed to be caused by all those "overweight" and "obese" people eating too much food. The assumption is not made specific anywhere on the page. It just *is*. "Fat is caused by eating too much and not exercising enough" is the truism that will not and cannot be questioned.

The pro argument is based upon privacy and personal responsibility. Balko essentially argues that making any kind of public health policy is leading Americans down a road to "socialized medicine."

Nowhere does he argue that fatness is simply a human characteristic. He is arguing that as long as he doesn't have to foot the bill, he will live and let die. He does not question the health and fat connection at all. He does not question the food and fat question at all. He assumes, like Brownell and Nestle, that being fat is bad for you and that overeating causes fat. He just doesn't think it is a public issue.

The con argument is based upon the social-problems claim generated by the war on obesity. Fat is bad. Overeating causes fat. Losing weight is good. Researchers, pharmaceutical companies, government policy-makers and street-level bureaucrats are responsible for finding a cure to help those who suffer from the illness of "overweight" and "obesity."

Even though they acknowledge that "humans are hardwired, as a survival strategy, to like foods high in sugar, fat and calories," and even though they admit "imploring people to eat better and exercise more" is a "failed experiment," Brownell and Nestle blame the food industry, the government, and the schools for not taking care of fat people and fat children.

No space is made in this either/or debate for multiple points of view. No one was asked to talk about simply accepting biology and demedicalizing fatness.

Balko is saying that fat people are responsible for their fatness, and therefore deserve whatever personal problems fatness causes them. He says, "Give Americans moral, financial and personal responsibility for their health, and obesity is no longer a public matter but a private one—with all the costs, concerns and worries of being overweight borne only by those people who are actually overweight." He concludes, "We're likely to make better decisions when someone else isn't paying for the consequences."

Balko essentially ignores a big part of the problem of being fat in the current cultural context. If being fat were truly a "personal" choice, then fat people could negotiate with their doctors, health insurance providers, and employers on the basis of their health rather than their size. Balko is pretending that the social aspect of the stigma/stereotype interaction doesn't exist.

Personal responsibility is impossible if a person isn't free to control her or his own body. Fat people cannot go to certain places without being harassed. Fat people are discriminated against in employment. Fat people are denied effective health care and health and life insurance because of their size.

Fat people cannot be personally responsible, because fat people are not free to be fat and healthy. These restrictions on their freedoms further exacerbate problems with their health, and the self-fulfilling prophecy is born.

Brownell and Nestle seem compassionate to the plight of the fat person on the surface, but they still have little respect for fat people. Like all supposed saviors, the anti-obesity researchers have an infantile view of those they claim to be helping. They argue that the food companies are taking advantage of poor fat people who are genetically predisposed to eating too much and gaining weight. They argue that these unscrupulous companies are creating fat people by marketing to kids. They argue that food companies put profits above people.

I am always amused at this form of salvation, because the diet industry, which supports much of the research done by people like Brownell and Nestle, often puts profits above people as well. Their argument encourages a diversified food industry with "diet" foods being marketed by the same people selling sugar, fat, and calories. Brownell and Nestle and their colleagues make it possible for the expansion of the market and the further exploitation of the same people they claim to be helping.

The either/or question implies that weight is a simple matter with simple solutions. The truth is that it is a complex phenomenon with a long social history that has made a number of things impossible to know.

I cannot know how much of my body weight is due to genetics and how much is due to a lifetime of dieting. I have relatives who are fat, but I probably have the largest BMI of any of my relatives. My older fat relatives worked in coal mines and on farms most of their lives. They probably never dieted, though they may have had lean times when food was scarce. They were physically active most of their lives. Their weights probably stayed steady, with the usual pound-or-two-a-year gain, until their 60s and the inevitable weight loss of old age.

I was fairly active most of my life until I got sick with lupus, but I have also worked in offices using my brain more than my brawn. I have lost and regained hundreds of pounds. I have yo-yoed up and down the scale repeatedly. I believe this history has contributed to my having a higher BMI than my relatives. I also believe that if I had never been on a diet and had been more physically active in my life, I still would have been fat—maybe not as fat as I am now, but certainly fatter than the conventional stupidity would want me to be.

It has taken a lot of effort to reclaim my appetite and my sense of satiation. I would be lying if I claimed that I had successfully done so. I have spent significant blocks of time in my life relearning what I believe should be natural cues. I am still learning.

I practice mindful eating when I can. Such eating is done attentively and nonjudgmentally, in the way Zen masters listen to their breath. I do not always practice this, however, and I have learned to be gentle with myself. I do not intend to make mindful eating a regimen the way I made dieting and exercise a stringent ruler over my time. Mindful eating is something I do to re-center myself when life gets hectic or when I feel flare-ups coming on. It helps. When I eat mindfully, I know my own hunger and my own fullness.

I have watched children eat, and they seem to know when they are hungry and when they are full. I am not sure if I will ever eat that naturally again. But it is those physical cues to which I try to listen rather than the public debate. So in a way, I will never know for sure if I am eating as nature intended me to eat.

Many people as fat as me often have problems with mobility. I have always walked or run slower than most other adults. When I was a runner, I was a long-distance runner, not a sprinter. I am shorter than most people are, and my stride length is short for someone my height. So going slower than others has been my plight in life no matter what I have weighed. In truth, my weight hasn't helped. Of course, neither has lupus or asthma.

A frequent argument raised to encourage drastic weight-loss measures for so-called morbidly obese people has been an argument regarding mobility. Indeed, there is no doubt that many of those few who have successfully lost weight are more mobile. I admit it is a tough argument to counter when you move slowly and your mobility is restricted. I can point to a number of factors, but I can't say with certainty that being fat does not restrict my mobility.

But I do have a theory. There *are* very large people in the world who are extremely mobile. They are strong. They probably have a lot of muscle mass, and they carry their weight well. Their strength increases their mobility. One explanation for much of the mobility problem of very large people might be found in social factors rather than biological ones. The root of these problems may be in the ways in which fat kids and fat young adults are taught to move their bodies.

Contrary to the conventional wisdom that the more fat you have, the less muscle you have and vice versa, most fat people have larger muscle mass than normal as well. It takes a lot of strength to carry weight, and moving around increases that strength.

Like any other human being, the more fat people use their muscles, the stronger their muscles become. This is one reason the fat suit is such a sham. As weight is gained, muscles are strengthened in everyday activities. You do not suddenly add 80 pounds of fat. You gradually gain fat and muscle over time. If you don't yo-yo diet, the gain normally is quite gradual.

So my theory is that if fat kids and fat young people were taught to strengthen their muscles instead of possibly diminishing them through weight loss, they would be more mobile and agile as they aged.

Socially, fat people are ostracized and alienated. They do not get to move around a lot without harassment. Walking or riding a bike in public is often met with jeers. Going to a private gym can be difficult because the physical spaces and personnel often do not accommodate larger people. Equipment that might assist larger people in muscle development is often not geared towards them.

I love weight training, but I rarely have used weight machines, especially lower body ones. I don't fit the machines that are usually found at a gym. This was true when I was thinner because I am short, and now it is also true because I am fat. My body shape just doesn't conform to the machine's parameters. So I use free weights, pulleys, and water resistance equipment.

Exercise is usually promoted as a means of losing weight rather than for its intrinsic benefit. Larger people often give up on exercise as useless when they aren't losing weight. They judge their progress by the numbers on the scale instead of the good feeling they get from the

Fat Olympians

The 2004 Summer Olympics were the first I had watched in several years. Their timing came at the end of my writing this book, and as such, I found myself acutely aware of body size and athleticism. That is probably why I noticed how many fat Olympians there were competing.

My favorite by far was Hossein Reza Zadeh, the Iranian weight-lifting gold medalist. Watching him lift a total of 472.5 kilos was amazing.

The 353-pound, 6'1" strong man had a style that entertained and warmed the heart. As he raised the barbells up to his chest and then over his head in the clean and jerk competition, veins bulged in his neck and face. He turned red with the strain. Sweat poured over his head. Would he make it? Would he break the record?

Barbells stretched out overhead with feet firmly planted— you knew the moment he had it, because a beautiful smile showed his accomplishment.

energy.

Exercise is also usually promoted as a task. A "no pain, no gain" attitude discourages many. Instead of playful and fun movement, exercise has become a chore, and it is a chore whose only payment is weight loss. Doing the chore and not losing weight is considered unrewarding.

My theory is simple. The mobility problems most larger people experience are a direct result of a lifetime of being limited by social, not physical, factors.

In the same way that dieting had all but destroyed my sense of hunger and satiation, ostracism and harassment had all but destroyed my body's strength, stamina, flexibility, and balance, as well as my sense of the playful fun of moving my body.

The smile would grow into laughter. Standing there with a world record 263.5 kilos extended above his head, Zadeh would laugh out loud and nod towards the cheering crowd. Then he would shout a large "whoop!" and put down the barbells. No translation needed. Everyone understood his pure joy.

When the movies depict Olympians competing on Mount Olympus, they choose the chiseled bodies made famous by Greek sculptures. But the return of athletes to Mount Olympus in the summer of 2004 featured hefty shot put throwers.

Even the usually detached announcer Bob Costas (a Greek-American) was obviously moved by the history of the moment. The Olympic movement has suffered in recent years, but in many ways it still represents the ideals of athleticism and competition. It is about striving not so much to defeat another as to push oneself to excel. It is about striving to push the human body to its limits to discover what those limits are.

Mount Olympus is often considered a grand symbol of what is best in sports, athleticism, and competition. What a

Finding friendly spaces in which we can move freely and safely is a difficult task for most fat people. We have learned through experience that public places come with certain dangers.

Even going to gyms, spas, and fitness centers can be a hassle. Other patrons and even the staff of such places can be insensitive to the feelings and needs of fat people. Injuries due to improper use of equipment that is designed for smaller people are prevalent, especially when staff are not trained in the specifications of the fitness equipment and do not inform fat people of those specifications.

My master's thesis was a participant-observation study of aqua-aerobics classes at a private health spa. I found that not only did other patrons regard the older and larger patrons as not having a "right" to the pool for their classes, but the staff was not supportive of the classes, and the physical layout of the pool area made the classes difficult to at-

joy for me to watch the return of games to Mount Olympus featuring bodies that looked more like mine than like the thin models so often touted as symbols of beauty and strength in our society.

Shot-putter Adam Nelson caught my attention because of the classy way he handled defeat. Regarded as a gold medal contender, he kept making mental errors, often stepping over the foul line in his efforts. He walked away with a silver medal, but the expectations had been higher for him. He made no excuses for his mental errors, although I believe just being at Mount Olympus might be distracting enough.

He stated emphatically that win or lose, he was experiencing a great deal of joy just being there. It was the end of his career, his last international competition. What a way to go.

Fat men, of course, are much more respected in sports than are fat women. But there were plenty of fat women athletes competing in 2004.

Gold medalist (2000) Cheryl Haworth began weight training at age 12. She is proudly fat and proudly strong. Her

tend. These barriers made it difficult for larger people to remain faithful to their routines.

Basically, having to deal with hostile territory takes all the fun out of movement, as it would for anyone. Because most of these businesses are set up to make money by discouraging attendance rather than encouraging it (by collecting monthly dues for services they do not have to deliver), not much effort is made to accommodate fat people in their efforts to exercise, even if they have weight loss as a goal.

In addition to this, our complaints of arthritis pain and other mobility-threatening conditions are often met with an admonition to lose weight rather than substantive treatment. This discourages us from going to doctors early in a disease process, making substantive treatment, when and if we finally do receive it, difficult to be effective. Thus, small problems that affect mobility become big problems because of the so-

---

parents never made her size or her eating habits an issue. In 2000 her coach, Michael Cohen, told Radiance magazine,

> At five-feet-ten-inches, and 290 pounds, Cheryl is at absolute peace with herself. Contemporary society has just about destroyed the self-image of young women. I coach women. I see my kids, at ages thirteen to nineteen, at constant war with themselves. Their archenemies are the mirror and the scale. Cheryl has no internal conflict. She's content, she's happy, and she's focused. She knows what she wants to do, which is totally unusual for a sixteen-year-old girl.

Haworth injured her shoulder in June and knew going into the Olympics that she would probably not repeat her Sidney performance. Her story got told often, however, and hearing it also gave me great joy.

The 2004 +75kg Clean and Jerk Weight-lifting gold medalist, Gonghong Tang, was slightly smaller than Haworth

---

cial attitudes of doctors and the stigma placed on being fat rather than the biology of fat itself.

While I cannot say with certainty that a world where fat people are encouraged to carry their weight well rather than be at war with their fatness would produce more mobile large people, I believe that it is worth trying. What we do know is that making exercise drudgery and connecting it to losing weight is not working on any level.

I also believe that in certain circumstances in our society, people *are* encouraged to carry their weight—and their fat—well. Football linemen are often very big men. They are not only tall and muscular, they have body fat. Their BMIs would qualify them for weight loss surgery in a New York minute.

These guys train hard. Their job is to hold the line and/or push it

---

and not quite as strong, but certainly the 5'8," 265-pound Chinese athlete defies the stereotypes of both gender and race.

Fat athletes competed in judo competitions, shot-putting, javelin throwing, weight-lifting, Greco-Roman wrestling, boxing, baseball, track and field, softball, and water polo. These women and men were strong and muscular and fat.

The Center for Consumer Freedom noticed the discrepancy between the war on fat and the celebration of these athletes as the world's best. In an August 16, 2004 article posted at their www.consumerfreedom.com website, the center used the opportunity to call our government to task for using the flawed Body Mass Index (BMI) as the basis for public health policies.

So should kayaker Joe Jacobi (Overweight: 5'7',' 165 lbs) worry about sinking? Should water polo star Tony Azevedo (Overweight: 6'1',' 193 lbs) enter the belly-flop competition instead? Does track star Maurice Greene (Overweight: 5'9',' 176 lbs) belong in the 100-meter waddle?

towards their goal line. They have to be quick off the count, but they don't have to run very far. They have to be strong enough to push other guys about their size out of the way to create holes for teammates to run through. They have nicknames like "Hog" or "Refrigerator."

Over the years, their training has become more sophisticated. They lift weights. They probably lift large objects like cars as well. The point is that no one says to *them* "you can't be fat and strong."

Some of them are encouraged to lose some weight, but rarely are they expected to conform to the conventional recommendations of BMI. Going from 350 pounds to 330 pounds might make you a better lineman, but if you lose down to 180 pounds, you are off the team.

In baseball, hard-hitting designated hitters are often fatter than the norm, sometimes approaching the conventional "morbidly obese"

I would go one step further. These fat athletes demonstrate that fatness and fitness are not opposites. Fat people cannot only be fit, they can excel in sports.

While paying attention to these athletes, I also came to appreciate how different bodies were better suited for different activities. Height made a difference in many sports. One of the women divers had originally wanted to be a gymnast. As she grew up, however, she became too tall for the sport and turned to high board diving because her gymnastic training helped, as did her newly developed height.

All the athletes were at the mercy of their genetics, to some extent or another. Training could only enhance what nature had endowed.

When I think about the struggles of all of us against the tyranny of stigmatizing differences, I believe that the Olympics offered us a valuable lesson. As a reluctant fat warrior in the war on fat people, my only desire is to live in a world where I can be allowed to be the best person I can be.

That is not too much for any human being to ask.

range. While there is a movement afoot in baseball to demand that players lose weight, they are often not pushed if they work out and play hard.

My favorite story about a fat player being harassed by management in baseball is the story of pitcher David Wells in his 1998 season with the New York Yankees.

Wells is a big guy, probably "obese" by conventional standards. He was in the starting rotation of the Yankees, and after a particularly bad outing, manager Joe Torre publicly took him to task for being too fat to pitch.

Without losing any significant weight, upon his very next start, on May 17, 1998, David Wells went into the history books as one of only a few players who have pitched a perfect game. In fact, only one other Yankee has ever pitched a perfect game in the entire history of the team.

To my knowledge, Torre never publicly discussed Wells' weight again.[9]

Fat athletics exist, and some fat people, mostly men, are encouraged to carry their fat well rather than lose it. When I began weight training again last year, I asked my trainer to teach me to lift weights "like a man."

Most women are taught to use weights as added aerobics aids. They do high repetitions with low weights and rarely increase their lift weights. I train twice a week and I push my muscles to exhaustion when I do. This builds strength. When I am consistently strengthening my muscles, I find that my stamina gets better as well. Stronger muscles make it easier for me to breathe.

It is a slow process for me because of lupus, fibromyalgia, and asthma. It is also a slow process because I am 46 years old. But I've been doing this for nearly a year now, and I can feel the difference in my stamina, strength, flexibility, and balance.

I believe there could be more fat athletes if fat people were encouraged to carry their weight well rather than lose weight.

The biological and genetics arguments that are used to dismiss the athletic prowess of fat people are reminiscent of arguments used against people of color in the history of the major sports.

In their essay, "The Negro Leagues and the Contradictions of Social Darwinism," son and father philosophers Alex and Rob Ruck outline the "scientific" arguments that were used to exclude African-Americans from sports at the end of the 19th century. These arguments were drawn mostly from Herbert Spencer's understanding of racial inequality as being a matter of "survival of the fittest" rather than a matter of imperialism and racism. There are some eerie parallels with discussions of fat and fitness:

> Most whites contended that African Americans were genetically inferior at sport, lacking the emotional equilibrium, endurance, and psychological makeup necessary for athletic achievement. Many believed that black boxers were plagued by weak stomach muscles, unable to absorb a blow. Nor did they think that African Americans had the stamina to run long distances or perform well late in a game. Such beliefs were used to justify the near-total exclusion of blacks from the mainstream of sport...Their absence reinforced assumptions of black inferiority. Segregation also meant that black athletes had little chance to disrupt philosophies of white superiority. They could not win if they could not compete, at least in the short run.

Fat kids are picked last at recess and in phys. ed. Fat kids are told to lose weight before they can join a team or compete in a sport. Fat kids grow up to be adults who believe they have no ability for sports and that it is their fatness that keeps them out of the game.

Since they are not encouraged to compete, are not trained to be athletic, and are treated with contempt when they try to join in, there are few opportunities to develop fat people as athletes. This kind of segregation becomes a self-fulfilling prophecy.

No one is born a fully trained athlete. Social circumstances help determine who will and who will not develop into an athlete. Telling fat people to go home and lose weight before they can come out and play sets up a vicious cycle that only ends up supporting the stereotypes about fat being bad.

Genetics is both a curse and a blessing to fat people. It is evoked in arguments asserting the inferiority of fatness *and* in arguments for fat acceptance.

The adaptation argument (not unlike the "primitive" label given African Americans) is that fat people are relics from an age of starvation. What was once an asset, the ability to store fat efficiently, is now said to be dangerous and harmful in the age of plenty. While genetics may explain a lot of the variation of people in terms of size, it is a big jump to assume that natural selection is the cause of people getting fatter than they are "supposed to be." The "caveman" scarcity explanation smacks of social Darwinism more than science.

Even Charles Darwin himself argued that variations in human beings were more a result of social and cultural changes than biological ones. Adaptation at the species level is not the same as adaptation at the individual level.

Social Darwinism attempted to divide human beings into groups that just do not make sense in biological terms. Some of us may be more genetically disposed to being fatter than others are (or have darker skin or different eye shape and so forth) but we still have more in common with our fellow human beings than we have differences. Discussions of adaptation and difference are based more often in culture than in biology.

When thinking about weight training and fat athletes, I became interested in sumo wrestling. Sumo is a sport based in the martial arts. In feudal Japan, members of the samurai class were regarded as elite soldiers, capable of great feats in battle. Within the samurai class were the sumo, men of great weight and height who were essentially the marines of the samurai. They were the first to fight in combat. Like linemen in American football, the sumo's job was to push the combat line back and open spaces for their comrades to move through.

The sumo warrior was considered among the bravest of soldiers. They were afforded servants who ensured that they were given enough food to maintain their size and their strength. They trained long hours.

Sumo wrestling matches are a remnant of the martial art of pushing people out of the way. Matches only last about eight seconds, though the ceremony before a match can be quite elaborate and take as much as 15 minutes. The object of the match is simple: The first guy to knock the other guy out of the ring or down on the floor wins. But this is not as easy as it seems.

I've watched a number of sumo matches on late night ESPN (a blessing of insomnia). The biggest guy doesn't always win. The wrestler has to have a knowledge of balance and a center of gravity that helps him judge where best to push his opponent. Smaller men sometimes have the advantage because their center of gravity is lower, making them harder to push down or out.

By the time the match starts, each of the sumo wrestlers has developed a plan. When the match starts, they both execute their plans, and the one who has the best plan wins. There is rarely time to change strategies, so they have to know what they are doing before they begin.

If the enemy in the war on fat is ideas and if the battleground is the dominant culture, then the sumo wrestler provides a great symbol for fat warriors. I like to think of fat warriors as being on the front lines of a battle that will change economic and social paradigms.

The North American economy is currently dependent upon most people in our society being dissatisfied with their possessions, their bodies, and their lives. We are sold problems, and then we are sold to advertisers as potential customers, and then we are sold half-baked solutions to those problems. If a time came when we were satisfied with our possessions, our bodies, and our lives, there is a fear that we might stop spending.

I think one of the most telling moments regarding consumer culture was in October 2001 when Federal Reserve Board Chairman Alan Greenspan told Americans that the best way to respond to the terrorist attacks of the previous month was to return to the malls and spend money on Christmas shopping.

Fear of fat is part of the waste and over-consumption that fuels an economy that increasingly seems to benefit the few at the expense of the many. A radical acceptance of fat bodies and a commitment to strengthen fat people by opening up spaces where people can just be fat without harassment or pressure will provide a space for all bodies to be strong and for all kinds of people to be accommodated.

I am coming to see my struggle to live as a fat person in a world that wants me to be thin in light of the sumo warrior. Fat people like me who strive to live unapologetically fat, to care for the body nature gave us, and to be comfortable within our own skins, are on the front lines in the war on *all* bodies.

The extent to which we are successful in challenging and changing cultural beliefs about fat, about ideal bodies, about health, about

---

Closet Optimist

(written summer solstice 2002)

I am a closet optimist. Now I'm about to write a bunch of stuff that will make one think otherwise, but the truth is, deep in my soul, I am an optimist.

This is not a popular position among most liberal, progressive, activist, academic, intellectual, artistic types with whom I hang out. Most of these people are known for the sorrow with which they identify and the things against which they stand. Anti-fill-in-the-blank is not usually an optimistic position because it becomes important for the anti-whatever to convince others that things are B-A-D, bad. After the convincing, maybe something could be done, but they never seem to get past the convincing part.

It is not that I'm not against a lot of what is going on in the world. The fact is that a lot of what is going on in the world is against me.

This week alone:

- Southwest Airlines wants to charge me double because they can't be bothered to build a seat big enough for me. Jay

---

economics, and about difference is the extent to which people of all sizes will have room to be themselves.

In order to fight this war, we may have to push some treasured ideals and sacred truisms out of the ring. Accepting the largest among us may make room for an army of samurai warriors who no longer worry about how well they stack up against an impossible ideal.

If we come to understand that fat is not inherently bad and that fat people can be strong, perhaps pseudo-science and looksism will no longer threaten the health and welfare of all people.

Ending the "war on obesity" is conceptually simple: Just stop fighting it. Make "obesity" an antiquated "disease" that gets left in the

Leno decided that it would be fun to further the cause of fat hatred as a shill for SWA by making fat jokes under their sponsorship.

- The Library of Congress has decided to make hobbyists pay for broadcasting on the Internet, and the website that provides the streamline for our radio show may try to charge us for royalties on our own material because complying to the LOC record keeping is prohibitively expensive and it would just be easier to assume everyone is playing someone else's music. A minimum charge would mean not only that we would be paying the Recording Industry Association of America (RIAA) for original work that we produced ourselves, but since our listening hours are so low, we will be subsidizing the larger sites with more listening hours, so we would, in effect, be paying a higher royalty than those sites that actually play RIAA music.

- Canada's Society of Composers, Authors, and Music Publishers (SOCAN) is pushing for a similar levy in Canada

history books like "dropsy" or "neurasthenia."

Ending the war on obesity is not easy, however. It requires nothing less than rethinking our culture's view of bodies, health, and beauty. That rethinking could start with fat people carrying their weight well.

However it begins, the war must culminate with appreciating and celebrating people of all sizes.

---

that may eventually kill community radio, thus taking out my only other outlet for being heard.

- My leftist sympathies are pushing me further in the "enemy of the state" category and make me ever more leery of what I write on the Net as "security measures" around the G-8 summit (the annual meeting of the heads of state or government of the major industrial democracies) are exaggerating and inciting police to hurt more people in the name of fighting terrorism and protecting freedom.

It isn't just the politics. I have poor friends who can't find jobs, and sick friends who are recovering from illness, injury, and surgery, and sad friends who are going through transitions.

And not being long in a new country, Canada, I don't have many local friends. I am often lonely in my politics, my cultural constructions, and my daily life.

Add to this that I feel guilty most of the time. I heard on the radio today that a Jewish writer wrote that in order to survive in a concentration camp, one had to lie, cheat, steal, and compromise. "The best of us did not survive" was the quote given by a First Nations (aboriginal Canadian) writer, who went on to say that she "felt that way about the reservations as well."

I have survived a lot in nearly 45 years.

I have survived personal tragedies such as the death of a baby, the loss of a marriage, and the loss of several jobs.

I have survived a melanoma on my leg and pre-cancer cells

---

on my cervix and systemic lupus erythematosus.

I have survived violence and violations such as being molested as a child, having a gun pointed at me in a robbery, having stuff stolen from me in break-ins, seeing my husband assaulted by a supposed friend on my own front porch.

I have survived being accused and suspected, though never arrested, of "wrong-doing" without an explicit charge being levied. For example, I have been harassed by police or had someone call the police on me for being in the wrong neighborhood, wearing the wrong kind of clothing, driving the wrong kind of car, and having the ability and the audacity to speak my mind or "talk back."

I have survived jeers and bullying based upon how I look, and I have survived the internal voices that stay in my head years after events, telling me I'm not good enough, not pretty enough, not smart enough, just not enough—or sometimes, too much and not staying in my place.

A friend called me a coward yesterday because I backed out of a confrontation. Maybe I am. Maybe that is why I survived so long. Maybe I lied, cheated, stole, compromised too often. Maybe I should be dead now. Maybe the best of me has not survived these things.

Instead, I sit in relative paradise, surrounding by trees, mountains, flowers, and safe streets. Instead, I hold a Ph.D. and a relatively interesting and well-paying job. I am not completely satisfied with my life, but the quality of my problems certainly has increased.

I have felt survivor's guilt.

But the older I get, the less I believe the survivor's guilt story. I think the best of us are surviving even when we resort to cheating, lying, and stealing, or even cowardice, in order to survive. I did what I had to do, and I will continue to do what I have to do. I am not going to apologize for surviving, nor am I going to forget that my survival was not meant to be.

I am not supposed to be here, doing what I am doing, being who I am. I am supposed to be in my place.

Today is the summer solstice. For a person with lupus, this is one of the hardest days of the year, especially if the weather is particularly sunny, as it has been today. It is the longest day of the year. But is also a marker of survival, because I know that for another year I have survived the lengthening of the days and can now look forward to shorter days and less sunshine and therefore fewer flare-ups and less joint pain.

We often think that the end of something is a bad thing. We mourn endings. This comes from reductionist, dichotomous or linear ways of thinking. But if we take the time to look around us, we find that in nature the end of something is often the beginning of something else.

A sunset ends the day, but begins the night. Dawn ends the night in preparation for another day. When an old star explodes, it becomes a nebula, a nursery for a thousand more stars.

I spent today outside, mostly in shaded wooded areas on top of mountains or near streams. I saw an old tree stump that was probably from a tree over a thousand years old. It was about seven feet in diameter and half of it was rotting away from the weather and the bugs, but the other half had three large trees growing out of it. Where one large tree had stood for centuries now three trees grew, using the root system of the old tree. I sat for about half an hour just staring at this adaptation, this cycle of life.

When I got my Ph.D. last year, I went to a tattoo salon to celebrate. I now have a phoenix on my left arm. It is there to remind me that I, too, have risen from the ashes, many times over. I am an optimist because Mother Earth is an optimist.

Those in the world who would have me be their slave continue to try to strike me down, but my hope is that I will survive, even past the death of my body. That is why I write. That is why I make radio. That is why I continue to fight the good fight.

So I am outed now—I AM AN OPTIMIST.

Deal with it.

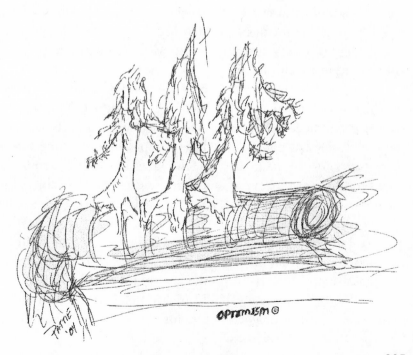

OPTIMISM

Knowing My Place

Some Concluding Thoughts

This book has been mostly biographical in nature, telling the story of how I changed my mind and my heart about fatness, and how fat acceptance has changed my life. But this book has also been sociological in nature, examining fatness and anti-obesity with the sociological eye I cultivated in graduate school. As I wind down writing, I want to pause, step back, and see the larger picture that made this book a necessary one to write for me and for the larger culture within which I live.

The act of writing this book has been an act of sorting out the ways in which my personal story has been and continues to be bound and connected to the larger culture. Like Alice, I wanted to see how deep the rabbit hole has gone. What I have found from working through these issues for the past 10 years, thinking and talking about these topics for the past three years, and from researching this subject more intensely for the past six months, is that the hole is deeper than I have ever let myself imagine.

The strong financial interests of the diet-pharmaceutical industrial complex ensure that many people stay motivated to ignore contrary voices and support efforts to promote weight loss. When I first heard the term "diet-pharmaceutical industrial complex," it made immediate sense. I cannot think of a better term for the intricate and complicated financial interests that surround anti-obesity research, products and policies. Other authors such as Laura Fraser in her book *Losing It* and Paul Campos in *The Obesity Myth* have done a fine job outlining who is in bed with whom. The term "complex" barely does it justice.

One of the more frustrating aspects of writing this book has been that the diet-pharmaceutical industrial complex grows constantly. A new medicine, study, treatment, or policy is announced if not daily, then at least weekly. As I write this final chapter in the summer of 2004, the latest addition to the complex is that U.S. Health and Human Services Secretary Tommy Thompson has changed Medicare and Medicaid policy to recognize "obesity" as a disease and to authorize payment for "effective" treatments.

In a fair world where truth was the test of government policy, I would not be that worried about Thompson's July 2004 testimony before Congress. No effective treatments of "obesity" actually exist, because long-term weight loss is rare and attempts to lose weight are often harmful. However, in the real world of politics and policy, this announcement means that more poor fat people will have their stomachs mutilated in an effort to lose weight, and more poor fat people will be guinea pigs for pharmaceutical treatments that are being rushed through safety assurance processes because of the supposed crisis nature of "obesity."

The only health improvement this decision is likely to create is an increase in the financial health of the physicians, surgeons, pharmaceutical companies, and other anti-obesity producers and providers who will cash in on this expanded market. Increases in Medicare and Medicaid payments go directly to the service providers, with only cursory considerations of whether the health of so-called beneficiaries is improved.

Like the Cold War reference implied in the term "industrial complex," these financial interests are so tied to fat being something to cure that I wonder if they would be excited if they *did* find a cure. They are making so much money and gaining so much prestige from the fight that I doubt they really care whether the health of fat people improves or not.

Exacerbating these financial interests is that the for-profit private medical system of the United States is built upon an authoritarian interaction between health care worker (expert) and patient (novice). Medical research remains mystifying to the general public. Words like "scientific," "statistics" and "studies" are considered magical in their ability to assert unproven statements as hard facts. Much of what patients know about medicine they learn from people claiming to be experts, whether they are practicing physicians or actors who play doctors on TV.

Arguments made by authority are problematic even if the authority is earned and well-informed. Those experts who have done their research, thought analytically about data, and drawn logical and rational conclusions from their observations do not need to argue from authority. They make their cases based upon reviewing methodology and opening their research reports to scrutiny. If science happened in a social vacuum, then medical information would be scrutinized and patients would be able to trust the recommendations made to them.

While medical consumers are savvier than they were 40 years ago, the basic authority of medical health professionals and medical researchers remains intact. "Studies have shown . . ." remains a powerful rhetorical device, justifying changes in behavior for most North Americans. But the nature of medical knowledge and the confusing and conflicting statements made by seemingly equally authoritative sources make assessing the truth value and usefulness of the words after the word "shown" next to impossible.

A great deal of damage has been done under medical authority. Physicians often prescribe "acceptable treatments" that endanger health, well-being, and life, telling fat patients that the risks are worthwhile, "for their own good." Perhaps more dangerous is that the lack of questioning of medical authority works its way up the chain, so to speak. Health care professionals rarely question what they read in major medical journals and pharmaceutical press releases. Public policy makers rarely question published conclusions found in major medical journals. Medical researchers rarely question previous published works found in major medical journals.

Major medical journals receive funding from pharmaceutical companies and other financial interests. In recent years, the editorial staffs of several of these major journals have changed policy regarding disclosure of funding sources, so that such potential conflicts of interest are not often noted. The entire medical research and treatment mechanism is so geared to adhering to the status quo on substantive matters and ignoring procedural considerations that once an inaccurate statement becomes axiomatic, it is quite difficult to challenge and revise. (Witness the proliferation of the inaccurate "300,000 deaths a year from obesity" statistic, which in 2004 was growing to 400,000 deaths per year. By late 2004, the figures had been shown to be calculated inaccurately and the revised estimate is 100,000, but even that estimate is fraught with problems.) Only the most drastic and deadly mistakes receive scrutiny, and often only after a lot of people have died or became ill or injured.

Scientific study, of course, is meant to be scrutinized and not meant to be based upon argument by authority. Scientists are taught methodology in order to ensure reliability and validity of their studies, not merely to credential the scientist. (Had they not been taught these issues, these issues would still remain, by the way.) But medicine is based almost squarely upon authority. The health care provider is expected to know things that the patient should not have to know in order to be healthy. The health care provider's credentials assist the patient in deciding who to trust and who not to trust. This tension between scrutiny and authority makes the current war on obesity particularly insidious.

I am often regarded as a cynic. I prefer to think of myself as a skeptic. In order to understand the contexts of one's life and the social nature of our interpersonal interactions, one must spend some time asking critical questions and refusing to accept every complete sentence one hears or reads as if it were divine revelation.

This book has a great deal of documentation in it. It also relies upon other sources of knowledge based upon, to name a few, emotional, empirical, analytical and existential precepts. Many academics believe that documentation and peer review constitute the best basis for grounding knowledge. I am skeptical of making this standpoint the supreme test.

Much of this book has questioned knowledge. How do we know

what we know? Many people accept their cultural knowledge as "givens." They rarely ask questions about their source of information. They see some sort of documentation like "studies show" or "scientifically" and they believe that the mere presence of the words ensures that the information is correct. Worse yet, many people hear something in conversation or in media and remember only what they hear, not where they learned it. The hearing of it makes it true.

I watch criminal justice documentaries upon occasion. Often as the story unfolds and we find out that the original person accused and/or convicted of the crime is found to be innocent, the family members of the victim refuse to accept the new evidence. Inevitably, they support the police or the prosecutor's first choice as the one who "did it." I am amazed at this phenomenon. It would seem to me that a family member would want the truth above all else. If DNA evidence shows that the original suspect isn't the killer, then wouldn't the family member be in the front of the line demanding that the police and prosecutor find the person who really committed the crimes?

The only explanation that I have for the family members clinging to the belief that the first person suspected of the crime is the criminal is that accepting the first information one hears as "true" is a deeply embedded part of our society (and, possibly, human nature). Most people believe that the first thing they hear is the correct information and that all other information after that must be tested against that first thing. This is a poor strategy. It leaves one open to all sorts of flim-flam artists. Con artists count on this phenomenon to fool their victims. The only defense against being conned is to examine critically what we know and how we know what we know.

Epistemology is a discussion or discourse addressing how one "knows" things and what sorts of "knowledge" can be found in various concepts. *Substantiation* is an effort to support one's arguments through some means of legitimation in order to convince one's listeners that what one is saying is true or meaningful. Substantiation makes use of all forms of epistemology, as well as raising, appropriately, the question of epistemology itself.

Documentation is only one form of substantiation. If this were not true, then observation, intuition, and innovation would be forgotten. But documentation should not hold a special status in the legitimation game. It is one form, not *the* form. Scientific knowledge is useful for many endeavors, and I recognize, rely upon, and appreciate the value of such knowledge. But that knowledge does not happen in a social vacuum. Giving scientific knowledge—and, indeed, the word "science"—magical powers must be viewed as quintessentially unscientific, if the word "scientific" is to be defined non trivially. Only a skeptical view of all documentation will lead to better knowledge. Only a recognition of the many ways our knowledge can be substantiated can lead to fuller knowledge.

Calls for documentation create a game that leaves many academic disciplines squarely in the throes of the status quo. Because academics often only accept what is published in particular journals and what has passed review by peers, knowledge production is slowed down and tends to support what is previously known. This has some advantages, but when bad ideas get into the system, it can lead an entire discipline astray. This happens more often than most academic disciplines want to admit. Some of what this book has outlined is the history of such bad information. Others have done a better job of outlining such histories.

The only antidote to this perpetuation of bad knowledge is epistemology. Discussions of knowledge and the production of knowledge are a necessary part of understanding truth. It is a rare and beautiful thing when an academic discipline takes the time to self-reflect upon its own tenets. Such a reflection is a necessary error-checking mechanism.

Of course, calls for documentation are often insincere in practice. They often reflect only a desire on the part of those who call for it for the persons they are addressing to shut up. There is a common, two-step rhetorical ploy that reflects this insincerity. In the first step, one calls for "documentation;" in the second step, regardless of the documentation provided in response, one rejects its sufficiency. There are a number of stock remarks serving the second step of this process that have become current. These include, "Well, that's just your opinion," and "Well, that's not an authoritative source." This approach, despite its paucity (as it begs the question of how the "documentation" game, meant to provide an antidote to arguing from authority alone, is substantially different from arguing from authority at all, and is pathetic in other respects), is pandemic in the academic and policy-oriented research circles I have frequented.

What this boils down to is very simple: Critically examine everything, no matter what authoritative reference is given. This book has been such a critical examination.

On one hand, the diet-pharmaceutical industrial complex controls a great deal of the information available regarding fat bodies. This information has been built upon axioms that few researchers and health care professionals question. Because the wrong questions are being asked and researched, the available information is biased towards a view of fat bodies as diseased. Because the questions that are being asked support the goal of the diet-pharmaceutical industrial complex (which is to promote weight loss treatments), these slanted studies will continue to be funded.

On the other hand, health care workers rely upon these sources of information for their initial training and continuing education regarding the latest treatments of the so-called disease "obesity" and related conditions such as diabetes, heart disease, and high blood pressure. The extent to which such educational exercises remain merely ritualized reading and repeating of information is the extent to which these axioms will remain in place.

It would be a mistake, however, to lay the pervasive cultural belief that fat is a disease singularly at the door of medicine and science. Making fatness a disease lies in a larger and more widespread belief that fat is ugly.

The extent to which fatness is regarded ugly in and of itself is the extent to which people will buy weight loss products. The language of science is used by the diet-pharmaceutical industrial complex, but the players in that complex are perfectly happy to use images, attitudes, and prejudices about fat people to promote weight loss.

Those images, attitudes, and prejudices serve a larger consumption-oriented economy that thrives on the dissatisfaction of consumers, making it imperative for consumers to remain critical of their lives and their bodies. Fear of fat not only drives consumers to try a vast array of mostly ineffective weight loss treatments, it feeds into an American mindset that says each person must purchase products in order to find health and happiness.

Operating in conjunction with consumption-oriented economics is the desire to create mass markets for products. The tendency in today's global economy is towards oligarchy, with only a few sellers providing standardized goods and services to a large audience. Media providers are in the business of convincing advertisers that they can reach those large audiences. Creating the image of a standardized body helps in standardizing the goods and services that serve those bodies. It also helps media providers convince advertisers that their audiences will buy those products.

The mass market is an enduring myth. I say "myth" because even with the frequent trend or fad, diversity still thrives. People come in all shapes, sizes, colors, and cultural backgrounds. People have varying needs, abilities, interests, talents, tastes, and desires.

Many people, however, are not confident in their bodies or their desires. Many people seek satisfaction from what they buy rather than from who they are. In a world where desire is commodified and sold to the highest bidder in the form of advertising, it is difficult to know if we want what we want because we want it, or because we were told to want it.

Vilifying fatness serves this standardization. In the world of popular culture, it is a given that everyone wants to be thinner. In the world of popular culture, it is a given that fat is unwanted. This means that in the world of popular culture, people will buy weight loss schemes. It also means they will buy clothes that make them look slim, spa vacations that make them feel thin, and cars that make thin people look good. In other words, thinness is just part of an entire image that is sold.

It is an image that costs a lot of money to create and maintain. Only a lucky few members of the population fit this image naturally. The remaining 99% have to do something in order to achieve the image. Most can't afford that effort.

A number of authors have made much of the fact that people of lower socio-economic status are fatter. Theories as to why this is true include differences in body shapes along ethnic lines, issues of access to nutritious foods and safe places to exercise, and perceived laziness among poor people.

Such theories make the assumption that anyone can be thin and anyone can be fat and that the difference between fat people and thin people is a simple matter of energy intake and expenditure. If this assumption were true, then a fear of fat would make sense. Why would anyone want to remain fat in a culture that treats fat people so poorly? Surely fat people are just too lazy or too unconcerned with their looks to do something about their image.

However, no one really knows why some people are fatter than others. It is true that energy intake and expenditure have something to do with weight, but clearly there are other factors. What if some people become fat no matter how hard they try to stay thin, and what if some people cannot gain weight no matter how hard they try? What if most people will gain only so much and are only able to lose so much?

I suspect that if we lived in a culture where no one tried to lose weight, people would naturally vary in size. I suspect that if we lived in a culture where no one tried to lose weight, individual weight would vary slightly depending upon activity and scarcity of food, but that variation would not be drastic. I suspect that if we lived in a culture where no one tried to lose weight, the fattest among us might not be as fat, and the thinnest among us might not be as thin.

But we do not live in a culture where no one tries to lose weight. We live in a culture in which the majority of us have been on a diet of some sort. We live in a culture where naturally fatter people use technologies to be thin.

My theory on the class differences in size is a simple theory: Richer people with natural tendencies towards fatness have the means to pass for thin. They spend their money on personal trainers, people to oversee what they eat, plastic surgery, and other technologies that keep them artificially thinner. It takes up an incredible amount of their time and resources, but it is part of the image they maintain. Even with this effort, many of them fail. The tabloids are full of reports of rich

A Tribute to My Dad, Ray Thomas

Given at Skycrest Baptist Church
Clearwater, Florida, on the occasion of his funeral
April 10, 1999
by Pattie Thomas

There are many ways to remember a life.

Obituaries reveal our place in world, where we were born, who survives us, where our memberships lie. The pastor read the obituary earlier of my Dad. I could add that his father was a coal miner in the mountains of West Virginia. He had eight brothers and four sisters. He loved his son-in-law and daughter-in-law like his own children.

We are often remembered by our accomplishments. Near the end, my Dad spoke of being a failure. He had few material rewards most of his life, and by the standards of a world obsessed by money and possessions, he may have been a failure. But in my eyes and in the eyes of all of you here who testify to his life by your presence today, he was a great success. He was a loving father, a hardworking and caring husband, a generous friend, and an honest business man. His riches were his right living, his friends, and his dry sense of humor. Children and animals were drawn to him, and as he told someone who visited him after he got sick, he liked people, he

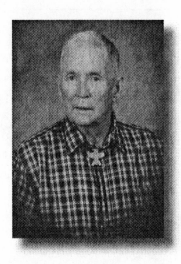

We are often remembered by our philosophy. My Dad's philosophy centered around front porches. He believed that America went downhill when people stopped building front porches, because they never got to know their neighbors anymore.

celebrities who lose weight only to gain more back.

This is not to say that poverty and fatness have a simple relationship in our culture. Fat people generally make less money than thin people, begging the question of which comes first. The war on obesity has increased discrimination against fat people by providing "legitimate" excuses for withholding jobs, health insurance, and other economic and financial benefits on the basis of size. I suspect that the differences of size between the rich and the poor will increase as well, as fewer people have the ability to buy the technology to pass for thin.

There are people and groups in this world who treasure nothing so much as one more excuse to discriminate. Having fat people continue to be blamed for their fatness would suit the selfish interests of these people and groups perfectly well. Being able to use the health excuse to cloak their discrimination in acceptable language only makes it more

needed people.

We are often remembered by the markers in our lives such as marriage, children, spiritual commitment, and life-changing decisions. My Dad married at the age of 25, had his first child at the age of 28 (me) and became a Christian at the age of 52. He was a very successful Volkswagen mechanic for 37 years, most notably at the old Sunoco on Drew Street. His decisions were not always successful, but they came from an honest attempt to live a decent life.

We are often remembered by the advice that we gave. The most memorable advice my Dad gave me was what I came to regard as "the college and the ditch" speech. From my earliest memory my Dad told me to go to college because "some day you will need a college degree to be able to dig a ditch." I took this to heart, maybe a little more than he wanted. There are some who believe I am a professional student. I will finish my Ph.D. next year. I wish he could have waited here to see me graduate, but I know he was proud. Of course, I think he worried that after all this schooling I'd only be able to get a job

appealing to encourage fat hatred.

The class dynamics of fatness intersect with race and ethnicity as well. Several studies have indicated differences in correlations between BMI and health conditions along ethnic lines. The diet-pharmaceutical industrial complex is increasingly targeting African-American women and Hispanic women. This can be seen in the increase of weight loss ads featuring testimonials from women of color, the increase of weight loss ads in magazines aimed at people of color, and the use of celebrities of color as spokespersons, such as Whoopi Goldberg's ads promoting SlimFast.

Dividing workers on the basis of their physical features has a long tradition in capitalistic economies. Such divisions have allowed employers to hire some workers at lower wages because of their ethnic backgrounds or gender. The strides made in the past 60 years discour-

---

digging a ditch.

We are often remembered by stories that we told or that others told about us. There were many of these that I will hold dear about my Dad. Last night I heard many stories from those of you who stopped by Moss-Feaster Funeral Home, and I'm sure we will all share more together. One of my favorites will explain a picture in the photo montage you may have wondered about.

About four A.M. one morning my Dad went down to the Sunoco station to open up and found an alligator sitting at the pump like it wanted a fill-up. A little shook up, he went across the street to call the police.

When he came back to wait for the wildlife people to show up, he found the alligator was gone. He said he was afraid they were going to accuse him of drinking or seeing hallucinations given the hour of the day. Frantically he searched for the alligator and found it about a half a block away. He waited for the authorities, watching both alligator and the road from the safety of his car.

aging racial discrimination and other visible differences have changed the labor market. Being able to divide workers on the basis of weight gives renewed power to employers in the employment relationship. Having access to the rhetoric of health instead of looks as the basis for these discriminatory practices hides that power relationship.

"Health," or rather, "health tendencies," has been used to justify discriminatory practices in the past. Women were considered physically inferior and at risk for injury at a number of jobs that they now perform skillfully. Mental and physical defects have been assigned to groups of people on the basis of how they look and their ethnic or cultural backgrounds to justify imperialism, slavery, and discrimination. If fatness is a natural variation of human bodies and not a health condition that is correctable through weight loss techniques, then the current war on obesity is yet another dismal chapter in a long history of hurting

Some newspaper reporters who knew my Dad and heard his name on the police scanner came to cover the story. The alligator made the *Clearwater Sun.* You don't see my Dad in the paper or in the picture we have put with the montage because, as he put it, "I was smart enough to hide behind the police car." He also concluded that it was a good thing he found the alligator again, because the newspaper might have reported his commitment to a mental hospital for seeing things.

He didn't just gripe, of course. He was quite kind to his neighbors, putting newspapers up on the porches of people who had trouble walking while he took his morning constitutional. I remember that when we were cooped up at JFK Middle School waiting for Hurricane Elena to pass, he was restless. To pass the time and deal with the boredom most people there played games or sat and talked. Not my Dad. He became a Red Cross volunteer and started sweeping in the cafeteria. He was a good neighbor no matter where his neighborhood happened to be at the moment. Perhaps this is why I chose to be a sociology researcher. I don't know, but I do think we need more front

people's life chances because of how they look.

I have argued in this book that the pairing of health and beauty in our culture serves to confuse what we consider good looks with good health and to make most of us feel bad about our bodies. The current rhetoric regarding poverty and fatness is helping to establish a pairing of wealth and beauty that makes thinness not only a health goal, but a status symbol.

During one of my games of *Flip* I came across a documentary about a woman who had a tummy tuck and breast enhancement after losing over 100 pounds. I'm not sure how she lost weight because I only watched a few minutes of the show. However, what I did hear was an amazing summary of the wealth, health, and beauty connection in pop culture.

porches and more friends like my Dad.

Finally, we are often remembered by our character. My Dad loved to tell the story of how an attorney told him that he would never have money because he was too honest. He concluded that this was a flaw in his character. I think it was his highest honor. The best word to describe my father was the word "decent." My Dad was a humble man who tried to do the right thing by everyone he met. Perhaps this cost him dearly at times, but it is the highest character, which I can only hope to achieve.

I almost missed getting to know my Dad. He worked a lot when I was a kid, and I didn't really know him well. When I was 16, I decided that it was important for me to have a relationship with the lump on the sofa that appeared every Sunday afternoon to sleep with football on the television and yell if anyone tried to change the channel. The way I got to know my Dad was to learn football. I succeeded in establishing a relationship with my Dad, and over the years it only got better. I'm happy to say that at the end of my Dad's life we talked and

After showing before pictures of her breasts and stomach (these were headless pictures of the specific body parts), the camera showed an "after" film of this large-breasted, small-waisted woman playing Frisbee with a child I assume to be her son. Her voiceover says, "It is easier to keep your weight under control after you have invested a lot of money to create a certain look."

I can think of no better description of the extent to which reshaping bodies, including weight loss, has become a preoccupation of the rich and famous and their wannabes.

In many ways, the wealth and beauty connection is reminiscent of Calvinism. According to the principles of Calvinism, the destiny of each person on earth is predestined, because God knows who the holy and who the sinners are before they are born. How do people on Earth know who has been chosen and who has not? According to their material blessings.

This line of reasoning allows for the justification of wealth as a sign of God's blessings, as the wealthy are obviously the chosen. If beauty is a sign of health and health is a sign of goodness, then the

laughed together and I felt close to him. I was indeed fortunate.

I wanted to tell you these things today because I need to remember and I want you to remember that Ray Thomas walked among us and touched us in ways that even he didn't fully understand. I want to honor this humble man who I was privileged to have for my Dad.

The Apostle Paul said that the "we only see through a glass darkly" in this life, so I don't pretend to know exactly what the next life is like. But in my imagination, my Dad is in heaven with an acre of land, a great big garden in the back yard and a big old wrap-around porch on the front. He's got a Cubs game on the radio, sitting on the porch, calling every animal he sees "Pluto," and waving at everyone with a little twinkle in his pretty blue eyes.

purchasing of thinness and beauty becomes a self-justification for both wealth and health.

The Calvinistic nature of the wealth, health, and beauty connection gives the diet-pharmaceutical industrial complex and health care workers a convenient resource in dealing with fat people. In the same way that rich people can justify their wealth and beauty (and goodness) on the basis of the ability to purchase symbols of health, fat people can be considered sinners by virtue of their inability to purchase the same symbols.

Being fat becomes the original sin. Only sacrifice and paying homage to these symbols offers the chance of salvation. Those successful at losing weight are saved by grace, predestined to be one of the chosen thin as foreseen by the anti-obesity dogma. Remaining fat or, worse yet, not trying to be thin, proves the sinner has rejected the dogma and will be condemned to a life of hell.

This is convenient because it allows those selling "obesity" treatments to blame the fat person if the treatments don't work. This is convenient because if a medical treatment causes harm to the fat person, it can be considered a price worth paying to be absolved of the sin of being fat. This is convenient because a successful treatment reflects well upon the provider of the treatment and not simply on the formerly fat person. The responsibility for weight loss rests upon the fat person, not upon the seller or the one who prescribes the treatment. The success story celebrates the treatment. Thus, an inevitable regaining of the lost weight signifies not a problem with the dogma, but with the sinner.

This is not to say that countervailing forces don't exist. The Internet has grown as a source of medical information, and is making it possible for patients to question medical practice and treatment.

In the summer of 2000, I did a survey of the *Journal of the American Medical Association (JAMA)* from 1990–1999, looking for articles, editorials, and letters that addressed changes in the doctor-patient relationship stemming from cyberspace. I found a few as early as 1990, but the number of articles escalated as the decade passed. Doctors reported anecdotally that patients were confronting them much more frequently with articles, treatments, and critiques from their own private research of their medical conditions.

But access to the Internet remains a class issue and a cohort issue. Younger and middle to upper class patients have better access to both private physicians and the Internet. Older patients and poor patients remain more at the mercy of the medical expert.

In addition, information from the Internet is not consistently good. The checks and balances placed upon medical research have a tendency to prevent new ideas from emerging and old ideas from being challenged, but the Internet has the opposite problem. Anyone with computer access to the Net can write anything they please about a subject, including medicine.

Of course, as this book and others have argued, medical research and so-called reputable sources of information can have serious defects even when they are regarded as legitimate. Sorting through information and finding the best ways to judge usefulness and/or truth value of that information is a problem older than cyberspace. How well medical consumers can sort through the vast array of information available and evaluate that information is a question for debate.

There is no doubt, though, that the Internet has changed the nature of the medical relationship. In my survey of *JAMA* articles, I found that early in the decade, physicians were reluctant to respond to patients who brought in their personal research. The questions asked were about compliance issues, and Internet-savvy patients were regarded as difficult patients. By 1997, the tone of the articles changed, with physicians looking to respond wisely to these patients, seeing them as cooperative and interested in their own health and welfare.

The common element, of course, was the evaluation of the patients' behavior solely in terms of the medical relationship, with an emphasis on how physician practice was impacted more than on patient health. The questions physicians asked were around assisting patients with sorting through information and learning how to use e-mail and web sites to increase their own practices and influence.

There are other good signs as well. A recent CNN report said that in 2002 75 percent of Americans felt that being "overweight" was not always a bad thing. This was up from 45 percent in 1985. Of course, CNN covered the story as a sign that fat Americans were letting themselves go, but the increase suggests the possibility of fat acceptance among those not content to let the corporate media tell them what to think.

While the health aspects of fatness are being questioned, the beauty aspects remain out of control. Almost every cable channel now has some form of a makeover show. Few of these shows concentrate on weight alone, but the same fuel that fires the anti-obesity sentiment in culture flames the belief that everyone could benefit from a makeover.

There is so much plastic surgery and Botox being used among celebrities, politicians, and rich people that I have visions of archeologists digging up the remains of people from the 21st century and concluding that we were cyborgs with silicon and mechanical parts built right into our carbon-based units. I doubt if there will be much evidence of weight loss surgery among the remains, but if such records survive, I can imagine the anthropologists in 3004 deciding that stomach-cutting rituals were a part of our religious practices.

Maybe I just watch too many sci-fi flicks, but the whole body-mutilation-to-improve-looks trend seems creepy to me. I sometimes watch celebrities on television and want to scream, "Am I the only one who thinks these people look unnatural? Am I the only one who *doesn't* think this makes them look better?"

It all has a *Twilight Zone* feeling. Of course, the answer is that plastic surgery has become a status symbol, and looking natural would not let others know about the symbol. It only raises status if others *know* about the effort and expense. Nature has little to do with the game.

Throughout the experience of writing this book I have had a gnawing feeling in the pit of my stomach. It comes from a dilemma I face by the mere act of writing about my experience as a fat woman.

On one hand, fat people rarely get to talk about fatness. It is important that fat people speak about their experiences. One of the ways that stereotypes are maintained is through the silencing of those stigmatized. On the other hand, a fat person writing a book about changing culture could lead readers to the conclusion that it is the responsibility of fat people to change the stigma placed on fat people.

Many of the street-level bureaucrats who work with fat people

understand the stigma placed upon fat people. Some of these bureaucrats, like the doctor who tried to talk me into weight loss surgery, use
the stigma to encourage weight loss. Some of these people understand
that the stigma is unfair, but they spend their efforts on helping fat
people cope with the stigma, with little attention to those people who
repeat the stereotypes.

*It is not the responsibility of the people who suffer under the oppression
of a stigma to change stereotypes.* It is the responsibility of those who
practice bigotry and repeat the stereotypes to change the stereotypes
and the stigma.

I know this dilemma cannot be resolved. Such is the nature of
culture and, most especially, language. The dilemma depends upon
people being easily divided into two categories: fat and fat-hater. These
are convenient categories when discussing prejudice, bigotry, stigma,
stereotypes, and oppression. But these convenient categories tend to
break down when examples of them are sought in the "real" world.

All humans have some body fat. All people carry fat on their
bodies; some just have more than others. Zero percent body fat would
kill you. Body fat is needed to maintain a balance of chemicals in
your body. This is one of the reasons no plastic surgeon has developed
liposuction treatments that will make really fat people thin. Removing
body fat is extremely dangerous when done in large amounts.

Putting people in oppressed and oppressor categories regarding a
natural process like fatness can become problematic quickly. The anti-
obesity researchers would have you believe your BMI puts you in one
category or another. But categories are often arbitrary and fuzzy.

I have spent most of my life since the age of 11 making some kind
of weight loss attempt. I have written volumes of journals with my
body measurements, my feelings when I eat or don't eat, lists of what
I have eaten with the nutritional content of every morsel, how far I've
run, how many reps I've done, and so forth. I have made notebooks full
of graph paper with charts of my weight and/or measurements and/or
dress sizes to track my progress. I still could probably accurately name
all the calories, fat grams, carbohydrate grams, fiber content and so-
dium content of most of the foods I see without looking up anything.

I was obsessed with food, fat, and my size for a very long time, and it has been an effort to let go.

The scale is a perfect example of how this obsession has manifested itself in my life. I stopped weighing myself when I stopped dieting. I had to do so. If I continued to note my weight, I would have continued to obsess over what I ate.

I have weighed myself only one time since that decision. When doctors' offices insist on weighing me, I usually talk them out of it. I make them give me a medical reason for doing so. When they do convince me they have a legitimate reason, I stand on the scale backwards and tell the nurse not to tell me the number.

I see scales in a number of places. Malls have scales. Health food stores have scales. Most gym dressing rooms have scales. Public bathrooms have scales. People's homes I visit have scales. Every time I encounter a scale, I literally have to talk myself out of weighing.

For nearly 30 years I weighed myself every time I used the bathroom. If I saw a scale, I mindlessly jumped on it "just to see." Now, I have to remind myself how squirrelly that number makes me. I have to remind myself how truly meaningless that number is.

One morning at my acupuncturist's office about 18 months ago, I had to use the restroom before I left. I was barefoot because I had not fully changed from my session with the doctor when I needed to use the facility. I felt light after the treatment. I was relaxed. Next to the toilet was a metric scale. As I sat there, I began to wonder how not dieting had affected my body. I began to wonder what I weighed.

I began a debate in my brain that sounds silly when I write it out, but it was a heated discussion in practice:

"Wouldn't it be nice to tell everyone that I lost weight from not dieting?"

"That's silly; I stopped dieting because my weight was irrelevant."

"But I feel so light today. I know I've lost weight. I feel so energetic."

"I guess it couldn't hurt anything to know. Why should I be so afraid of the scale? Maybe this is the next step. Maybe I should be able to know my weight and not care. This will be good for me."

I weighed myself, and it was higher than I thought it would be. I had not really gained much weight, but I certainly had not lost weight.

The simple act of weighing changed my entire perspective.

Author Geneen Roth in her book *Feeding the Hungry Heart* calls the scale "Judge Detecto" because most of us let the number on the scale judge us morally. The lower the number, the more "right" we are. Changes in the number create changes in our mood.

After weighing that morning, all the light, airy feeling drained from my body. I had to convert the reading in kilograms given me by the scale to the equivalent in pounds, so it took me a minute to do the math. Instead of enjoying the health and well-being that acupuncture had brought me, I was obsessively calculating and recalculating the conversion in my brain.

I couldn't believe I had gained weight. My mood turned dark. The scale had been my judge, and I felt the weight of its verdict months

Scales

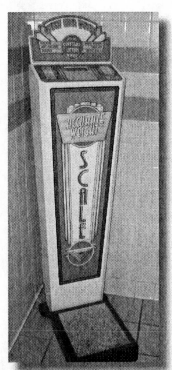

I recently saw a scale in the women's room at a truck stop that I thought had weight in perspective: "Exact Weight & Lucky Lotto Numbers."

Of course, the charts were available to let you know if your "exact" weight was "lucky" enough to be "ideal." What a day it could be to have an ideal weight and win the lottery at the same time!

While I was taking this picture, a woman walked into the room and smiled at me. I laughed and said I thought the scale was silly.

after deciding that it wasn't a relevant indicator.

It literally took me days to talk myself out of going on a diet and/ or going out and buying laxatives and diuretics, just to "lose a little." This emotional struggle took place even though I had decided and still solidly believe that weight is largely irrelevant to health and is a poor indicator of well-being.

The tyranny of the scale is a powerful force in this culture. Most people weigh themselves on a regular basis. It amazes me that, even in size acceptance circles, people give their weight in precise terms, as a constant. In actuality, weight is always imprecise, and the reporting of a single number belies that reality.

Most people weigh more after they eat a meal than they do when they wake up. Most people retain and release excess body fluids over the course of a week. Most people lose a little when they are more

She totally missed my explanation.

"I weighed on that scale last night," she exclaimed. "I don't think it's accurate at all."

"Not what you expected," I said half-heartedly, thinking that I was ending the conversation.

"There's one at the mall," she exclaimed, "that I think is right. It seems to be consistent, anyway. The one at the doctor's office is all over the place. I hate weighing there."

"I never weigh myself anymore," I say, trying to steer the conversation.

She would not have it. She listed at least five more scales she knew about and how they stacked up against each other.

I couldn't have asked for a more poignant example of the tyranny of the scale. Even fun scales like this one.

I didn't play the lotto that day.

I didn't weigh that day.

I figure I saved $1.25.

active and gain a little when they've been sedentary.

None of us weighs a single weight all the time, no matter how much Weight Watchers would have you believe you are "maintaining." Weight fluctuates. Actually, height fluctuates as well, but most people don't obsessively measure their height on a daily basis.

I suffer from lupus. Lupus is an autoimmune disorder. Normal processes in my body trigger immune responses and turn my body's natural defense system on itself.

My hands hurt nearly every day of my life. They hurt me when I type, like I am doing right now. The fluid between my joints remains inflamed most of the time. This makes my hands swell and my joints ache. It is the feeling most people get when they have the flu, because one of the defenses against a virus is to heat up different fluids in the body warm enough that the virus can't thrive. My immune system doesn't understand that there is no virus right now. It thinks that sunshine and halogen lights are viruses. It thinks the typing motion of my hands is a virus.

In some lupus patients, the immune system attacks cells in the heart, lungs, kidneys, or liver as if they were viruses. With an autoimmune disorder, the immune system can be so screwed up that it kills the body while trying to protect the body.

The current predominant view that body fat is bad is like an autoimmune disorder. It is like health care turning on itself. People who claim to care about health are treating normal variations in human bodies as if they are diseased and in need of a cure. The cures are killing people or, at least, destroying their health. Like lupus, fighting fat in the name of a disease called "obesity" is health care taking all of its defenses against disease, injury, and disability and turning those defenses against otherwise healthy people.

When an obesity researcher or a Surgeon General says "Join me in the war on obesity," he or she means that people need to lose weight and/or be thin in order to be healthy. When *I* say to you, "Join me in the war on 'obesity,'" I mean that people need to forget about the "disease" named "obesity" and understand that weight is a fairly poor indicator of health, and that in any case those who would make such a "condition" a priority of any health care system that exists cannot be indulged.

We will all be healthier when we stop making a natural part of our bodies a disease. Attempting to "cure" obesity is hurting a lot of people needlessly. Like all witch-hunts, it is wasting time, money and effort that could be used for more productive endeavors.

I started out writing a book about my story, about how over the past 10 years I have come to accept myself as I am, including my fatness. I started out writing a book about how finding beauty in fat bodies and finding strength in fat bodies has made me more comfortable in my own skin. Giving up dieting and learning to eat and exercise for my health rather than for my weight has led me to a better place personally and professionally. This book should be ending on a happy note.

But the truth is that I needed to write this book whether anything changed in the culture or not, and whether the writing of the book led people to hold those practicing bigotry accountable for fat hatred or not. I realized that if I want to pursue a life of creativity, I had to face this most pervasive and influential part of my life.

Goffman called stigma a "spoiled identity," and being treated horribly by so many people for so many years has certainly spoiled much for me. I am a well-educated person who has traveled a lot of places and met a lot of people. I enjoy writing, reading, photography, filmmaking, dancing, drawing, astronomy, traveling, and exploring the world around me. Yet, there have been long periods in my life when I have been afraid to leave my house, and when I have been lonely beyond endurance.

I have wasted a lot of time and a lot of my time has been wasted for me. My health is permanently damaged by what I have come to believe are the serious effects of my extensive, desperate and drastic attempts to lose weight.

I have missed much while I've been worried about my weight, my calorie intake, and my dress size. I know that I will never be the person I could have been. I have to live with that. And I am angry about that.

I am angry that for my most of my life researchers have known that diets do not work, and that in fact diets mostly make people fatter and unhealthy.

I am angry that while I was being taught "the scientific method" in school, the politics of the diet-pharmaceutical industrial complex were claiming to be scientific about my body while breaking all their own rules and ignoring their own data.

I am angry that no one warned me that I might be damaging my health by trying to lose weight. In fact, I was told exactly the opposite. I was told that *not* trying to lose weight was the source of all my problems.

I am angry that for my entire life physicians and other health care workers have been willing to tell me anything, whether it was true or not, and especially if it served their selfish interests, to get me to lose weight. I have been told that if I didn't lose weight, I would not be able to walk by the time I was 40. I have been told that if I didn't lose weight, I would get breast cancer or cervical cancer. I have been told that if I didn't lose weight, I would die by the age of 50 from a stroke, heart attack or diabetes. I have been told that if I didn't lose weight, I would have arthritic symptoms and fatigue indefinitely. I have been told that being fat caused my asthma. I have been told that being fat caused lupus. I have been told that being fat caused common colds.

I am angry that every counselor, clinical psychologist, social worker, or psychiatrist I have encountered as a client told me the proof that I was emotionally unstable was that my body was fat. I have come to believe that like physicians, mental health workers will say just about anything in order to motivate their clients to lose weight, or at least to motivate them to keep coming back and paying for sessions to figure out the hidden reasons for not losing weight.

I have been told that trying to lose weight would make up for my being raped at the age of five. I have been told that trying to lose weight would cure marital problems. I have been told that trying to lose weight would cure depression. I have been told that trying to lose weight would help me heal from losing my baby son.

I am angry that despite giving my time and money to a number of political causes, no one in the political spectrum stands up and says it is part of their platform to fight fat stigma.

I am angry that while I marched for women's causes, I was being given dieting advice from my "sisters."

I am angry that while I contributed to organizations fighting social economic injustices such as unequal food distribution and over-consumption of the rich at the expense of the poor, the leaders I supported were going on talk radio shows announcing that fat people like me were symbolic of how Americans over-consumed.

I am angry that every liberal in the country is jumping on the "save the fat kid" bandwagon, and that whole new generations of kids are facing the fat-bashing horrors of my childhood and adulthood as a fat person.

I am angry that the Surgeon General of the country in which I was born and of which I am a citizen has decided to demonize bodies like mine by comparing them to terrorists who fly jets into skyscrapers, blow up children on school buses, and poison air systems with deadly gases. I was a kid who worked hard in school, stayed out of "trouble" for the most part, and grew up to be a hard worker, willing to do more than a few things to better herself. I should be considered the all-American girl. But instead, I am being painted by my government officials as a drag on a virtually nonexistent "public health care system," while my so-called society refuses to employ me fully, extend me health care under any circumstances, or provide me with a decent wage, all because of how I look.

I am angry that I cannot leave my house without thinking about the spatial dynamics of where I'm going. Will I be able to sit in the theatre? Will I be charged extra for the plane seat? Will there be chairs without arms at the restaurant? Will I be able to fit in the restroom? Will I have to fold my arms and legs into uncomfortable positions in order to make myself smaller so I can fit into a world not designed for people like me?

I am angry that the act of taking up space in the physical world is regarded as radical and intrusive.

I am angry that even though there is room for everyone in this world, everyone is not invited.

I am angry that every single piece of entertainment I seek out, every advertisement to which I am exposed, every newspaper or magazine I read, every form of media I consume is colored by a view of bodies like mine as being bad.

No one ever asks me what I want. No one ever asks me what I think. No one ever asks me what feels comfortable, successful, or happy. Instead, I am told that if I only would try to lose some weight I could be happy, joyous, and free. I am told that I could have been someone important if I had lost weight. I am told that I would have been well-liked, had lots of boyfriends, and made good grades if I had tried to lose weight. I am told that if I were thin I'd be beautiful, rich and popular. I am told that because I am fat I am lazy, stupid, dirty, and ugly.

Being told without being asked is a sure sign of stigma. The idea that I would even begin to know my own body, my own satisfaction, my own mind, or my own heart is beyond comprehension in this system of thought. The thought that people with bodies like mine are a market segment that should be accommodated is lost in this system of business. I am fat, and that is apparently the only important fact about me in this culture.

Being fat means people can be rude to me without recourse.

Being fat means people can ask me highly personal medical questions even if they don't know me.

Being fat means kids can cry out epithets and laugh behind my back or to my face without being scolded by their parents, or, for that matter, by me.

Being fat means I can be turned down for many jobs without any explanation.

Being fat means that even when I get a job, other workers can harass me at will.

Being fat means that even though I have a Ph.D. and a portfolio a mile long, the first thing, and often the last thing, anyone notices about me is that I am fat.

I can't really find the words for the pain, anger, and loneliness I feel when it comes to the ways my fat body is depicted in popular culture. But of course, if I could really say those words, thousands of people would simply assume that weight loss would cure the pain, anger and loneliness.

On top of the anger is the frustration of never really knowing for sure if my social relationships are genuine or tainted. Laughter from the table next to me, stares on the street aimed in my direction, or dirty looks as I pass by evoke fear in me, but except for the most blatant of cases, I am never sure if laughter, stares, or dirty looks are really aimed at me. Even if there were situations where I could be sure these actions were aimed at me, I could not be sure they were aimed at me because I was fat. Am I just over-sensitive? Am I so war weary that I am hypervigilant? Certainly, that possibility can be raised by anyone caught treating me this way.

My identity is spoiled by anti-obesity fervor. I can tell my side of the story, but I cannot escape the spoilage. Until being fat is acceptable in this culture, I will have to deal with this in one form or another every day of my life. I pay and have paid and will continue to pay the price for this nonsense.

A fat woman happy with her body is a dangerous thing in the current culture. I know that writing this book will most likely bring me more grief. Being satisfied with a fat body flies in the face of several powerful interests that benefit from the belief that fat is bad. I am in the awkward position of hoping that this book is read by a lot of people and wishing that I won't have to deal with any more negative consequences of being fat and smart in this society.

There is a part of me that would just love to go live in Alaska or the Yukon with my husband and a bunch of dogs and sheep and stay as far away from people and North American culture as I can. I have to admit that I may yet do that if the dominant paradigm about my body doesn't change soon.

It is tiresome to live with the stress of this stigma. I often need to escape in some way to keep up my strength and perseverance. But escaping is difficult in a world in which we are constantly bombarded with messages about fatness, dieting and bodies.

One day, after ignoring all of the Atkins low-carb signs on our way back to the electronics department in a major discount depart-ment store, my husband picked up a Palm organizer that had a "diet" feature among the many calendars and scheduling devices available. The diet feature was a list of the nutritional values (fat grams, carb grams, vitamins, calories) of over 800 foods.

Keeping strict records of what we eat is now, it appears, considered as important as keeping appointments and keeping track of our accounts. My husband points out it also appears to be more urgent than including, within any product in the same price range, a "memo" feature that allows entries of sufficient length to permit a user to record a coherent thought.

This latter observation raises the issue of whether those who produce such technology have simply decided that those of us who are expected to consume such technology are to play the diet game to the exclusion even of writing.

I'm left with the question: Why should a fat person like me write a book like this? Why should I become a warrior in a war I did not start and do not want to fight? The answer lies in my optimism about the nature of culture.

Culture changes. Every book that is published, every show that is televised, every radio program that is aired, every newspaper article that is read, every play that is staged, every economic transaction that is made, every law that is passed, every person that is befriended, every enemy that is defeated, every single interaction between two or more people that takes place changes culture in some way. Culture is the sum total of all these micro-level events, and something is always being subtracted, added, divided, or multiplied. Culture changes.

Even if I do run away to the Outback some day and live with the wolves, my action will change culture. Whether it is a small ripple or a big splash, we are all connected to each other, and what we do does make things different to some degree or another, if only by the effect it has on the context in which future decisions and events transpire.

That is the good news and the bad news of culture. On one hand, as sentient actors in culture, we have a will that we exert, and that exertion changes things. On the other hand, so does everybody else, and some people's wills have bigger effects. So we are both powerful and powerless.

I do not know if this book will be a big splash or a little ripple. I have no control over whether someone will read this and decide that fat people have serious problems that would go away if they just lost weight. I have no control over whether someone will read this and realize that every single word of fat hatred (including the word "obesity") adds to the fire that consumes and hurts people.

But I do know that speaking with my voice and sharing my knowledge adds to the possibility of real change in the culture. Writing this book has given me strength. Only time will tell what effect it has on the rest of the world.

Culture will change because it is always changing. Because of that fact, I will remain the optimist, and will continue to be the reluctant warrior, taking up space.

Resources

The following resources are listed under category headings based upon the themes of this book. This is by far not an exhaustive listing. I am happy to report that there was just too much stuff out there to create a comprehensive guide. In addition, more is being created every day.

I tried to include things that were influential in my thinking or were recommended by people I respected—and it should be noted that several of these people made it quite easy to follow their recommendations by listing resources on their websites and in their own books which I shamelessly co-opted. I tried to include some things that I do not necessarily endorse, but feel would be important for anyone wanting to understand these themes to explore; therefore, these are recommendations for further study and not for further confirmation of my ideas or opinions. I tried to weed out things that were not easily available anymore. I tried to include different kinds of media, such video, audio, website, magazine and books, within each category, though it was not possible to include all forms of media in each category. I also tried to pick things that did not require a graduate degree in the topic in order to understand them.

I use the words "I tried" because I'm not sure I succeeded completely on any of these criteria. Still, what follows should stimulate thought and further personal research into these topics, and ultimately that is my goal. My apologies to all the good things I missed—I know there are many.

One final word: I did not try to document all sides of these categories. Specifically, I felt no need to document the other side of the "war on obesity."

Since there is a news item or new product almost every day that "attacks fat" in some way or another, I felt that anyone wanting to learn more about that side of things need only watch television, read a news service, or surf the 'net. One of the byproducts of stigma is that the side of the story of the stigmatized rarely gets a comprehensive hearing. So, since they are not fair, nor balanced in their reporting, I felt that it was time to tip scales of justice a bit in fat people's directions.

Advertising and Consumption

Can't Buy my Love: How Advertising Changes the Way We Think and Feel. Jean Kilbourne (1999). Touchstone.
> Explains advertising and its effects on culture and our self images

Commodify Your Dissent: The Business of Culture in the New Gilded Age. Thomas Frank & Matt Weiland, Eds. (1997). W. W. Norton & Company.

Enchanting a Disenchanted World: Revolutionizing the Means of Consumption. George Ritzer (2004). Pine Forge Press.

Killing Us Softly 3: Advertising's Image of Women. Jean Kilbourne (2000). Media Education Foundation.
> Latest in a classic series of videos examining how women are portrayed in advertising and media.

No Fat Chicks: How Big Business Profits by Making Women Hate Their Bodies and How to Fight Back. Terry Poulton (1997). Carol Publishing Group.

No Logo: Taking Aim at the Brand Bullies. Naomi Klein (2000). Picador.

Slim Hopes. Jean Kilbourne (1995). Media Education Foundation.

The Making of American Audiences from Stage to Television, 1750 to 1990. Richard Butsch (2000). Cambridge University Press.

The McDonaldization of Society. George Ritzer (2000). Pine Forge Press.

Anti-Dieting

Afraid to Eat: Children and Teens in Weight Crisis. Frances M. Berg (1997). Healthy Living Institute.

Eating Well, Living Well: When You Can't Diet Anymore. Glenn Gaesser & Karen Kratina (2000). Wheat Foods Council. 10841 S. Parker Rd., Suite 105, Parker, CO 80134 http://www.wheatfoods.org/.

Fat is A Feminist Issue. Susan Orbach (1979). Berkley.

Fat Talk: What Girls and Their Parents Say about Dieting. Mimi Nichter (2000). Harvard University Press.

Fed Up! Liberating Ourselves from the Diet / Weight Prison. Terry Nicholetti Garison with David Levitsky, Ph.D. (1993). Carroll & Graf.

Feeding on Dreams: Why America's Diet Industry Doesn't Work And What Will Work for You. Diane Epstein & Kathleen Thompson (1994). Macmillan Publishing Co.

Feeding the Hungry Heart. Geneen Roth (1982). Bobbs-Merrill Co. Inc.

Healthy Weight Network
http://www.healthyweight.net

Resources, information and research on weight and eating issues.

Hugs International
http://www.hugs.com
Information on nondiet approach to health and wellness for both health professionals and lay public.

Killing Us for Our Own Good: Dieting and Medical Misinformation
Dawn Atkins
Music by Cosy Sheridan (The Losing Game)
Body Image Task Force
PO Box 934
Santa Cruz, CA 95061–0934
Video covers success/failure rates of dieting, possible side effects of weight loss, theories of weight and metabolism, manipulation of medical research, effects of discrimination, and ways to effect change.

Living in a Healthy Body (1995). Krames Communications.
1–800–333–3032.
15-page pamphlet in consumer friendly language promoting lifestyle change rather than weight loss. Good teaching tool.

Making Peace With Food. Susan Kano (1989). Perennial Currents.
A self-help text and workbook for chronic dieters of all sizes and eating-disorder sufferers.

Moving Away from Diets: New Ways to Heal Eating Problems & Exercise Resistance. Karin Kratina, Nancy King & Dayle Hayes (2003, 1996). Helm Publishing, Texas.

Nourishing Connections
http://www.nourishingconnections.com/
Website dedicated to promoting intuitive eating.

Overcoming Overeating. Jane R. Hirschmann & Carol H. Munter

(1998, reissued). Fawcett.
  Promotes natural eating.

Setting the Record Straight
  http://www.wheatfoods.org/
    Book and kit on fad diets.

Staying Off the Diet Roller Coaster. Linda Omichinski (2000). Hugs International.
  Strong support for your diet-free lifestyle.

The Dieter's Dilemma: Eating Less and Weighing More. William Bennett & Joel Gurin (1982). Basic Books.
  Good for doctors and other health professionals who are still recommending weight loss diets. Explains why diets are obsolete and discusses setpoint theory.

When Women Stop Hating Their Bodies: Freeing Yourself from Food and Weight Obsession. Jane Hirschmann & Carol Munter (1997). Fawcett Books.

Women Afraid to Eat: Breaking Free in Today's Weight-Obsessed World. Frances M. Berg (2001, 2000). Healthy Weight Network.
  Practical guidelines for healthy change in weight and eating issues.

Women's Campaign to End Body Hatred and Dieting
  http://www.overcomingovereating.com/

Beauty and Body Image

200 Ways to Love the Body You Have. Marcia Hutchinson (1999). Crossing Press.

A Book about Girls, Their Bodies, and Themselves. Cordes, Helen (2000). Lerner Publications Company.

A New Look at Adolescent Girls: Strengths and Stresses.

American Psychological Association
750 1st ST., NE
Washington DC 20002
202–336–6031
bfreeman@apa.org

Adios, Barbie: Young Women Write about Body Image and Identity.
Ophira Edut (1998). Seal Press.
http://www.sealpress.com

Am I Thin Enough Yet? The Cult of Thinness and the Commercialization of Identity. Sharlene Hesse-Biber (1997). Oxford University Press.

Beanpole. Barbara Park (1983). Knopf.

Beauty Bound. Rita Freedman (1986). Lexington Books.

Bodies Out of Bounds: Fatness and Transgression. Jana Evans Braziel & Kathleen Lebesco, Eds. (2001). University of California Press.

Body Image Health
Kathy Kater
http://www.bodyimagehealth.org/
Website resources to promote healthy body image and size acceptance.

Body Image Task Force Newsletter
Mary Atkins, Director
PO Box 934
Santa Cruz, CA 95061–0934
408–426–1821
Quarterly newsletter

Body Image Workbook: An 8-Step Program for Learning to Like Your Looks. Thomas F. Cash (1997). New Harbinger Publications.

Body Outlaws: Young Women Write About Body Image and Identity.

Ophira Edut (2000). Seal Press.

Body Positive
http://www.thebodypositive.org
Multi-media approach to promoting Health at Every Size. Excellent materials for young people.

Body Talk: The Straight Facts about Fitness, Nutrition, and Feeling Great About Yourself. Ann & Julie Douglas (2002). Maple Tree Press.

Body Wars: Making Peace with Women's Bodies. Margo Maine (1999). Gurze Books.

Building Blocks for Children's Body Image
Marius Griffin
The Body Image Task Force
PO Box 360196
Melbourne, FL 32936–0196
http://home.earthlink.net/~dawn_atkins/children.htm

Exacting Beauty: Theory, Assessment, and Treatment of Body Image Disturbance. J. Kevin Thompson, Leslie J. Heinberg, Madeline Altabe, & Stacey Tantleff-Dunn (1999). American Psychological Association.

Fat History: Bodies and Beauty in the Modern West. Peter N Stearns (1997). New York University Press.

Fat: The Anthropology of an Obsession. Don Kulick & Anne Meneley (2005). Tarcher.

Girl Power in the Mirror: a Book about Girls, Their Bodies, and Themselves. Helen Cordes (2000). Lerner Publications Company.

Healthy Body Image: Teaching Kids to Eat and Love Their Bodies Too! Kathy Kater. (1998, 2005). National Eating Disorders Association.

http://www.nationaleatingdisorders.org
Curriculum for grades 4–6. Revised in 2005.

I Like Me! Nancy Carlson (1988). Viking Kestrel.

Liking Myself. Pat Palmer (1997). Impact Publishers.

Little Girls in Pretty Boxes: The Making and Breaking of Elite Gymnasts and Figure Skaters. Joan Ryan (2004). Warner Books.

Love Your Body Campaign
National Organization for Women's Foundation
Women's Health Project
http://www.nowfoundation.org/issues/health/whp/

Making Weight: Healing Men's Conflicts with Food, Weight, Shape & Appearance. Arnold Andersen, Leigh Cohn & Thomas Holbrook (2000). Gurze Books.
Issues for boys and men.

Never Too Thin: Why Women Are at War with Their Bodies. Roberta Seid (1989). Prentice Hall Press.

No Body's Perfect & No Body's Perfect Journal. Kimberly Kirberger (2003). Scholastic.

Phat Camp
Phat Camp
c/o Nomy Lamm
3540 N. Southport, #346
Chicago, IL 60657–1475
morethanjustphat@yahoo.com
http://www.morethanjustphat.com/
Fat positive, body positive experiences designed for youth and adults to learn about living in and loving their bodies.

Reviving Ophelia: Saving the Selves of Adolescent Girls. Mary Pipher (1994). Putnam.

Revolting Bodies?: The Struggle to Redefine Fat Identity. Kathleen Lebesco (2004). University of Massachusetts Press.

Revolution From Within: A Book of Self-Esteem. Gloria Steinem (1993). Boston: Little Brown & Company.

Survival of the Prettiest: The Science of Beauty. Nancy Etcoff (2000). Anchor.
> An examination of the assertion that preferences for beauty are genetic rather than culturally based.

The Beauty Myth: How Images of Beauty Are Used Against Women. Naomi Wolf (2002). Perennial.

The Body Project: An Intimate History of American Girls. Joan Jacobs Brumberg (1997). Random House.

The Truth About Body and Beauty. Kaz Cooke (1998). W.W. Norton & Company.

People. Peter Spier (1980). Doubleday.

Real Gorgeous: The Truth about Body and Beauty. Kaz Cooke (1996). W.W. Norton & Company.

Bullying

Bully Busters
> http://bullybusters.org

Bully in Sight: How to Predict, Resist, Challenge and Combat Work-place Bullying. Tim Field (1997). Success Unlimited.

Bully Online
> http://www.bullyonline.org
> A United Kingdom site that addresses a number of bullying issues.

Bullycide: Death at Playtime. Neil Marr & Tim Field (2000). Success Unlimited.

Bullying Prevention Program
http:www.colorado.edu/cspv/blueprints/model/programs/BPP.html

History of UK National Workplace Bullying Advice Line
http://www.bullyonline.org/workbully/worbal.htm
The advice line is now defunct, but this history includes statistics regarding the prevalence of bullying in schools and workplace from a United Kingdom perspective.

Kidpower
http://www.kidpower.org
Self-defense, conflict resolution and anti-bullying resources.

Post Traumatic Stress Disorder: The Invisible Injury. David Kinchin (2004). Success Unlimited.
Includes bullying as a form of trauma.

Commerce and Economics

Diet for a Small Planet. Frances Moore Lappe (1991). Ballantine Books.

The Ample Traveler
http://theampletraveler.com
Website dedicated to promoting universal access in the travel industry.

The Cluetrain Manifesto: The End of Business as Usual. Rick Levine, Christopher Locke, Doc Searls & David Weinberger (2001). Perseus Books Group.

The Clustering of America. Michael Weiss (1988). Harpercollins.

The Nature of Economies. Jane Jacobs (2001). Vintage Canada.

The Overspent American. Juliet B. Schor (1998). Basic Books.

Critique of Obesity Science

An Interview with Paul Campos. Pattie Thomas (2004). *Big Fat Blog.*
http://www.bigfatblog.com/columnists/archives/001240.php

Big Fat Lies: The Truth about Your Weight and Your Health. Glenn
Gaesser (2002). Gurze Books.
Complete reference for scientific data supporting the concept
that metabolic fitness is more important than fatness and
can be achieved without weight loss.

*Consequences of Dieting to Lose Weight: Effects on Physical and Mental
Health.* Simone A. Frency & Roberty W. Jeffery (1994). *Health
Psychology.*

Fat is Not a Four-Letter Word. Charles Roy Schroeder (1992).
ChronMed.

Fitness, Not Fatness, Is the Issue. Steve Blair (Fall 1999). *Well
Newsletter.*
http://www.speakwell.com/well/199_fall/articles/cooper_
watch.html

Health at Every Size Journal
Editors: Wayne Miller and Jon Robison
Gurze Books
PO Box 2238
Carlsbad, CA 92018
1–800–756–7533

Is It Necessary to be Thin to be Healthy? Glenn A Gaesser (2003). *The
Harvard Review.*

Jon Robison, Ph.D.
http://www.jonrobison.net/index.html

This website promotes Health At Every Size in the context of a holistic approach to health

Losing It: America's Obsession with Weight and the Industry That Feeds It. Laura Fraser (1997). Dutton.

Making the Case for Size Acceptance
Deborah Burgard. Ph.D.
    http://www.bodypositive.com/argument.htm

Obesity and Socioeconomic Status: A Complex Relation. Albert J. Stunkard & Thokild L.A. Sorensen (Sep 20,1993). *New England Journal of Medicine.*

Paul Ernsberger, Ph.D.
    http://www.cwru.edu/med/nutrition/ernsberger.html
    Remarkable work regarding the genetic components of fat bodies.

Psychosocial Consequences of Weight Cycling. Susan J. Bartlett, Thomas A. Wadden, & Renee A. Vogt. (June 1996). *Journal of Consulting and Clinical Psychology.*

Rethinking Obesity: An Alternative View of Its Health Implications. Paul Ernsberger & Paul Haskew (1987). Human Services Press. Well documented rebuttal to the old NIH Panel pronouncement that obesity is a "killer disease." Originally published as a special issue of the *Journal of Obesity & Weight Regulation.*

Separating Fact From Fiction—In Matters of Size and Weight
Carol A. Johnson, M.A.
    http://www.largelypositive.com/Pages/MythFact.html

Show Me The Data: Blog
    http://www.showmethedata.info/
    Source of discussions on latest obesity research from a Health at Every Size viewpoint

The Center for Consumer Freedom: Promoting Personal Responsibility and Protecting Personal Choice
> http://www.consumerfreedom.com/
>> Financed by food and restaurant interests, this website contains considerable information regarding the problems with obesity science.

The Obesity Myth: Why America's Obsession with Weight is Hazardous to Your Health. Paul Campos (2004). Gotham Books.

The Spirit And Science Of Holistic Health: More Than Broccoli, Jogging, And Bottled Water; More Than Yoga, Herbs, And Meditation. Jon Robison & Karen Carrier (2004). Authorhouse.
> A critique of health promotion, challenging health care professionals to think about well-worn medical models and to truly promote health and well-being.

Theoretical Underpinnings for Women's Health. A. B. McBride & W. L. McBride (1981). *Women & Health.*

Thrifty Genes and Human Obesity: Are We Chasing Ghosts? Per Bjorntorp (2001). *Lancet.*

Culture and Society

A Sociological Tour through Cyberspace
> http://www.trinity.edu/~mkearl/
>> A comprehensive source of all things sociology.

Contexts
> University of California Press/American Sociological Association publication
>> New York University
>> 4 Washington Square North, #345
>> New York, NY 10003
>> 212–998–8296
>> Fax: 212–995–4714

editor@contextsmagazine.org
http://www.contextsmagazine.org/
> American Sociological Association's most accessible journal.

Cultural Construction Company
Pattie Thomas, Ph.D. & Carl Wilkerson, M.B.A.
> http://www.culturalconstructioncompany.com
>> Admittedly our website, but we believe it offers a nice set of everyday sociology resources.

Cultural Criticism: A Primer of Key Concepts. Arthur Asa Berger (1994). Sage Publications.

Cultural Resistance Reader. Stephen Duncombe, Ed. (2002). Verso. Perhaps the most fascinating collection of cultural writings available.

Culture of Fear. Barry Glassner (2000). Basic Books.

First Person, Plural
Pattie Thomas., Ph.D. & Carl Wilkerson, M.B.A.
> http://fpp.culturalconstructioncompany.com
>> Radio Show, aired 2002–2004. Descriptions and transcripts of the broadcasts are available on the website.

From Modernism to Postmodernism: An Anthology. Lawrence E. Cahoone, Ed. (1995/2003). Blackwell Publishers.

Introducing Cultural Studies. Ziauddin Sadar, illustrated by Borin Van Loon (1998). Totem Books.
> Comic book format with dense material, great introduction to cultural studies in Europe, the Commonwealth and U.S.

Introducing Sociology. Richard Osborne, illustrated by Borin Van Loon (1999). Totem Books.

Comic book format with dense material, great introduction to sociology.

Is Science Multi-Cultural?: Postcolonialisms, Feminisms, and Epistemologies. Sandra Harding (1998). Indiana University Press.

Narratives in Popular Culture, Media, and Everyday Life. Arthur Asa Berger (1996). Sage Publications.

Never Satisfied: A Cultural History of Diets, Fantasies and Fat. Hillel Schwartz (1986). Free Press.

Postmortem for a Postmodern. Arthur Asa Berger (1997). AltaMira Press.

Singing Sociology
Minna Bromberg
minna@minnabromberg.com
http://www.minnabromberg.com/soc/soc.shtml

Sociological Snapshots 4: Seeing Social Structure and Change in Everyday Life. Jack Levin (2004). Sage Publications.

Sociology: Snapshots and Portraits of Society. Jack Levin & Arnold Arluke (1996). Sage Publications.

The Bust Guide to the New Girl Order. Marcelle Karp & Debbie Stroller, Eds. (1999) Penguin.

The Culture of Pain. David B. Morris (1993). University of California Press.

The Happy Mutant Handbook: Mischievious Fun for Higher Primates. Carla Sinclair, Gareth Branwyn & Mark Frauenfelder, Eds. (1995). Riverhead Trade.

The Onion Presents Our Dumb Century: 100 Years of Headlines from America's Finest News Source. Scott Dikkers, Ed. (1999). Three

Rivers Press.

> Parody at its biting finest. A sideways look at culture, society and history and funny to boot.

The Self We Live by: Narrative Identity in a Postmodern World. James A. Holstein & Jaber F. Gubrium (1999). Oxford University Press.

The Sociologically Examined Life: Pieces of the Conversation. Michelle Schwalbe (2004). McGraw-Hill College.

The Standard Deviants: Sociology, Parts 1 & 2. Ruth Westheimer (1999). Cerebellum Corporation.

> Videos introducing basic sociological concepts through skits, humor and interviews.

Disability and Chronic Illness

Abilities Magazine
> The Canadian Abilities Foundation
> 340 College Street, Suite 401
> Toronto, ON M5T 3A9
> 416–923–1885
> Fax: 416–923–9829
> info@enablelink.org
> http://www.enablelink.org

Ability Magazine
> 1001 W. 17th Street
> Costa Mesa, CA 92627
> 949–854–8700
> Fax: 949–548–5966
> http://www.abilitymagazine.com

Access Unlimited's Link Barn
> http://accessunlimited.com/html/link_barn.html
> Website providing resources for persons with disabilities.

Association for Applied and Therapeutic Humor
Karla Pollack, Executive Secretary
5 Independence Way, Suite 300
Princeton NJ 08540–6627
609–514–5141
FAX 609–514–5131
staff@aath.org
http://www.aath.org/

But You Look Good: A Guide to Understanding and Encouraging People Living With Chronic Illness and Pain! Wayne and Sherri Connell. IDA.
P.O. Box 4067
Parker, CO 80134
Booklet to help sufferers of invisible disabilities share information with family and friends

Crip Korner: A Place to Rest Your Wheels
http://members.tripod.com/~cripkorner/index.html

disABILITY Information and Resources
http://www.makoa.org/
The most comprehensive resource links for disability issues available on the web. "Makoa" is a Hawaiian word that means "courageous."

dizAbled
http://www.dizabled.com
Cartoon following the antics and accomplishments of wheelchair hero Leeder O Phobes—great humor in the face of adversity.

Good Days, Bad Days: The Self in Chronic Illness and Time. Kathy Charmez. (1991). Rutgers University Press.

Healing Well
http://www.healingwell.com/pages/

A website dedicated to bringing people with chronic illness together for support and sharing information.

Mainstream: Magazine of the Able-Disabled
http://www.mainstream-mag.com/

National Organization on Disability (NOD)
910 Sixteenth Street, N.W.
Suite 600
Washington, DC 20006
202–293–5960
Fax: 202–293–7999
TTY: 202–293–5968
ability@nod.org
http://www.nod.org

New Mobility
No Limits Communications Inc.
P.O. Box 220
Horsham, PA 19044
215–675–9133
Fax: 215–675–9376
http://www.newmobility.com

The Center for an Accessible Society
http://www.accessiblesociety.org/
This project ended in 2004, but the website is still available with archival information.

The Invisible Disabilities Advocate
P.O. Box 4067
Parker, CO 80134
http://myida.org
Website dedicated to helping people who have chronic illnesses that are not visible.

The Strength Coach
Greg Smith

Speaker—Syndicated Radio Host
877–331–7563
greg@thestrengthcoach.com
http://www.thestrengthcoach.com/
Inspirational speaker who "coaches" inner strength in spite of being born with muscular dystrophy.

World Association of Persons with disAbilities (WAPD)
4503 Sunnyview Dr., Suite 1121
Post Office Box 14111
Oklahoma City, Oklahoma 73135
405–672–4440
Fax: 405–672–4441
http://www.wapd.org

Eating Disorders

Academy for Eating Disorders
http://www.acadedis.org

After the Diet Newsletter
A Better Way Health Consulting
PO Box 11985
Glendale, AZ 85318–1985
623–486–0737
http://www.afterthediet.com

Association of Anorexia Nervosa and Associated Disorders (ANAD)
PO Box 7
Highland Park, IL 60035
847–831–3438
http://www.anad.org

Body Wise Handbook
http://www.4woman.gov/BodyImage/bodywise.cfm

A booklet to help parents and youth workers identify eating disorders in adolescent girls

Eating Disorder Referral and Information Center
http://www.edreferral.com

Eating Disorders and Men
Ira M. Sacker
http://www.eatingdis.com/men.htm

Feminist Perspectives on Eating Disorders. Patricia Fallon, Melanie Katzman, & Susan Wooley (1994). Guilford Press.

Food Fight: A Guide to Eating Disorders for Preteens and their Parents. Janet Bode (1997). Aladdin Paperbacks.

GO GIRLS! (Giving Our Girls Inspiration & Resources for Lasting Self-Esteem)
http://cart.nationaleatingdisorders.org/curr_main.asp
12-week media literacy curriculum. Focuses on enhancing self-esteem and training to empower savvy media advocates who can impact current media messages related to body image.

Good Answers to Tough Questions about Weight Problems and Eating Disorders. Joy Wilt Berry (1990). Children's Press.

Gurze Books
PO Box 2238
Carlsbad, CA 92018
800–756–7533
http://www.gurze.com.
Catalog, specializes in eating disorders books.

How Did This Happen? A Practical Guide to Understanding Eating Disorders. Institute for Research and Education (1999). Health-

System.

For coaches, teachers, parents to help them identify and help adolescents with eating disorders.

How the Namuh Learned to be Content with Who They Were. Kathy Kater (1999). Author.

2497 Seventh Avenue East, Suite 109
North St. Paul, MN 55109

A metaphorical children's story. Also included in Kater's book *Real Kids Come in All Sizes* (see the "Fat Kids" resources category), and as Lesson 2 in the revised edition of Kater's *Healthy Body Image: Teaching Kids to Eat and Love Their Bodies Too!* curriculum for upper elementary age children, published by the National Eating Disorders Association in fall 2005 (see the "Beauty & Body Image" category). A freestanding version of the story and its discussion questions can be purchased by sending a check for $5 to the author at the address above.

Mirror Mirror

http://www.mirror-mirror.org

National Eating Disorder Information Centre (Canada)

College Wing 1–211
200 Elizabeth St.
Toronto ON M5G 2C4
Canada
416–340–4156
http://www.nedic.ca

National Eating Disorders Association (US).

Seattle, WA.
www.nationaleatingdisorders.org

Resources, information on treatment and prevention.

Something Fishy

http://www.something-fishy.org

Studies in Eating Disorders—An International Series: The Prevention of Eating Disorders. Walter Vandereycken & Greta Noordenbos (1998). The Athlone Press.

Your Dieting Daughter: Is She Dying for Attention? Carolyn Costin (1997). Brunner/Mazel Publishers.

Fashion and Style

Ample Crocheters
> http://www.ample-crocheters.org/
>> Website dedicated to promoting crochet patterns for larger people.

Ample Knitters
> http://ample-knitters.com/
>> Website dedicated to promoting knitting patterns for larger people

Beautiful Magazine
> info@beautifulmagazine.net
> http://www.beautifulmagazine.net/
>> New magazine serving women sizes 14+, scheduled to begin publication in summer 2005.

Belle: The Premier Magazine for Confident Full-figured Women
> 1–800–877–5549
>> For elegant, full-figured women, featuring African American women.

Grand Style
> http://www.grandstyle.com/
>> Website serving plus-sized women, including style, shopping and great resources for "living large."

Learning Curves : Living Your Life in Full and with Style. Michelle J. Weston (2000) Crown.

From the editor-in-chief of the now defunct *Mode* magazine.

Life Is Not a Dress Size: Rita Farro's Guide to Attitude, Style, and a New You. Rita Farro (1996). Chilton Book Company.

True Beauty: Positive Attitudes & Practical Tips from the World's Leading Plus Size Model. Emme (1996). G.P. Putnams Sons.

Fat Acceptance

Ama Menec
> http://www.amamenec.co.uk/index.htm
>> Sculptor—fat art work.

Ample Hygiene for Ample People. Nancy Summer. Willendorf Press.
20 page brochure, available through NAAFA bookstore.

Association for Size Diversity and Health (ASDAH)
> Claudia A. Clark, Ph.D.
> Counseling Center
> 320 Saddlemire Building
> Bowling Green State University
> Bowling Green, OH 43403
> caclark@bgnet.bgsu.edu
> 419–372–2081
> fax: 419–372–9535
> http://www.bgsu.edu/offices/sa/counseling/ASDAH.htm

BBW (Big Beautiful Woman)
> 4517 Harford RD
> Baltimore MD 21214
> 410–254–9200
> http://www.bbwmagazine.com

Big Adventures
> Scuba diving for the plus sized.

Liz Nickels, M.A., Psy.D.
http://www.BigAdventures.net

Big Big Love: A Sourcebook on Sex for People of Size and Those Who Love Them. Hanne Blank (2000). Greenery Press.

Big Dance
Lynda Raino
715 Yates Street
Victoria, BC. V8W 1L6
Canada
250–388–5085
bigdance@bigdance.org
http://www.bigdance.org/
    Fat dancing perfomances.

Big Fat Blog
http://www.bigfatblog.com
    Website examining media items surrounding size-acceptance. Includes discussions by members.

Big Options
PO Box 30094
Oklahoma City, OK 73140
Office: 405-732–6839
Fax: 405-732–3586
Bigoptionsnet@aol.com
http://www.bigoptions.net/
    Magazine and website with lots of information about organizations, reading materials, tapes, clothing stores.

Fernando Botero: Paintings and Drawings. Werner Spies, Ed. (1997). Prestel.

Bountiful Women. Bernell, Bonnie (2000). Wildcat Canyon Press.

Café Abundance
http://www.geocities.com/Paris/Cafe/7404/

Casa Gordita
>   Mary McGhee
>   http://www.casagordita.com/fatacc.htm
>   Website includes a great fat acceptance resource page.

Fat and Proud: The Politics of Size. Charlotte Cooper (1998). Women's Press, Ltd.
>   http://charlottecooper.net

Fat and Thin: A Natural History of Obesity. Anne Scott Beller (1977). Farrar, Straus & Giroux.

Fat Chance! Leslea Newman (1994). The Putnam & Grosset Group. A novel for ages 12 and up.

Fat Chance: The Big Prejudice. Rick Zakowich (1993). National Film Board of Canada.

Fat Chicks Rule! How To Survive in a Thin-Centric World. Lara Frater (2005). IQ Publishing.

Fat Dancer. Donna Allegra, in *Journeys to Self-Acceptance: Fat Women Speak.* Carol Wiley, Ed. (1994). Crossing Press.

Fat Girl Walking
>   http://www.fatgirlwalking.us/
>   Marsha is going to walk from San Francisco to New York in 2006 "to nurture the hopes of people of extraordinary size, disprove many myths about being fat, encourage people to get out and do something, and encourage people to put effort into their communities."

Fat Power: Thin May Be In, But Fat's Where It's At! Llewellyn Louderback (1970). Hawthorn Books.
>   The bible of the fat liberation movement, written by a co-founder of NAAFA. Available through NAAFA's bookstore.

Fat Underground Throws Weight Into Obesity War. Jane Wilson.

http://www.largesse.net/Archives/FU/LATimee.html.
Originally printed in the *Los Angeles Times* on January 8, 1976.

FAT!SO? Because You Don't Have to Apologize for Your Size. Marilyn Wann (1998). Ten Speed Press.
The quintessential text on fat acceptance.

FAT!SO? the website
http://fatso.com
Includes an online forum called Gab Café for discussing all things *flab*ulous

Fat: A Fate Worse Than Death? Ruth Raymond Thone (1997). Harrington Park Press.

Full Body Project
Leonard Nimoy
http://www.leonardnimoyphotography.com/7body.htm
Nudes photography by *Star Trek's* Spock—beautiful work.

Full Disclosure
James Stanley Daugherty (from 1999)
http://www.jsd.com/disclosure.html
Fat nudes

International Size Acceptance Association (ISAA)
P.O. Box 82126
Austin, Texas 78758
512–371–4307
Director@size-acceptance.org
http://www.size-acceptance.org/
Organization dedicated to promoting size acceptance worldwide.

Journeys to Self-Acceptance: Fat Women Speak. Carol Wiley (1998). The Crossing Press.

Largely Positive Newsletter & Groups
    Carol Johnson
    PO Box 17223
    Glendale WI 53217
    414–299–9295
    positive@execpc.com

Largesse, the Network for Size Esteem
    http://www.eskimo.com/~largesse
        A great website dedicated to size-esteem.

Live Large!: Ideas, Affirmations & Actions for Sane Living in a Larger Body. Cheri Erdman (1996). Harper Collins.
        Available from *Amplestuff:* 914–679–3316.

Lynne Murray
    Author of Josephine Fuller mysteries with plus-sized heroine.
    http://www.lmurray.com.
        At Large. Lynne Murray (2001). St. Martin's Press.
        A Ton of Trouble. Lynne Murray (2002). St. Martin's Press.
        Large Target. Lynne Murray (2000). St. Martin's Press.
        Larger than Death. Lynne Murray (2000). St. Martin's Press.

National Association to Advance Fat Acceptance (NAAFA).
    http://www.naafa.org
        Dedicated to human rights and improving quality of life, since 1969.

National Organization for Lesbians of Size
    http://www.nolose.org/

Nothing to Lose—Sane Living in a Larger Body. Cheri Erdman (1995). Harper Collins.
        Available from *Amplestuff:* 914–679–3316.

Overcoming Fear of Fat. Laura S. Brown & Esther Rothblum, PhD. (1989). Harrington Park Press.

Experts share personal and professional experiences of challenging fat oppression. An empowering guide for fat people and their supporters.

Pat Ballard

Author of romance novels and short story collection featuring big beautiful heroines.

http://www.patballard.com

A Worthy Heir. Pat Ballard (2004). Pearlsong Press.

Dangerous Curves Ahead: Short Stories. Pat Ballard (2004). Pearlsong Press.

His Brother's Child. Pat Ballard (2004). Pearlsong Press.

Nobody's Perfect. Pat Ballard (2004). Pearlsong Press.

Wanted: One Groom. Pat Ballard (2004). Pearlsong Press.

Plus Stuff… Your Primary Source for Living Fully

357 Tehama

San Francisco, CA 94103

Phone: 415-777-2158

Fax: 415-777-2260

Email: info@plusstuff.com

http://plusstuff.com

A combination of fashion catalogs, advice and news about fat, fat acceptance and related issues. It started in 2004 and claims to be "the first Internet lifestyle portal dedicated to the plus-size community."

Radiance Magazine Online

http://www.radiancemagazine.com

Scoot Over, Skinny: The Fat Nonfiction Anthology. Donna Jarrell & Ira Sukrungruang, Eds. (2005) Harvest Books.

Self-Esteem Comes in All Sizes: How to Be Happy and Healthy at Your Natural Weight. Carol Johnson (2001, 1996). Gurze Books.

> Encourages people above average size to accept themselves and focus on health and well-being rather than weight loss.

Sexy At Any Size: The Real Woman's Guide To Dating and Romance. Katie Arons & Jacqueline Shannon (1999). Fireside.

Size Acceptance & Self-Acceptance: NAAFA Workbook. National Association to Advance Fat Acceptance (1990). Author.

> Available through NAAFA book service: http://www.naafa. org. An introduction to the body of writing, theory, and policy that has evolved into NAAFA and the size acceptance movement. Includes chapters on health, fashion, employment, self-esteem, fat admirers, and activism.

Size Net

> http://www.sizenet.com
>
> The online library with the largest collection of articles about size- and self-acceptance. Covering many aspects as written by or about the fuller figured person.

Size Wise

> http://www.sizewise.com
>
> Website offering size-friendly resources and information.

The Afterlife Diet. Daniel Pinkwater (1995). Random House.

> Novel about fatness with a fat acceptance theme.

The Fat Girl's Guide to Life. Wendy Shanker (2004). Bloomsbury.

The ISAA Rapport

> P.O. Box 82126
>
> Austin, TX 78758 USA
>
> 512.371.4307
>
> http://www.size-acceptance.org/rapport/
>
> Archived podcast radio show produced by International Size Acceptance Association

The Strange History of Suzanne LaFleshe: and Other Stories of Women and Fatness. Susan Koppelman, Ed. (2003). The Feminist Press at City University of New York.

Wake Up, I'm Fat! Camryn Manheim (1999). Broadway Books.

What Are You Looking At? The First Fat Fiction Anthology. Donna Jarrell & Ira Sukrungruang, Eds. (2003.) Harvest Books.

Who Says Fat Isn't Sexy? Vanessa Feltz (1993). *Redbook.*

Without Measure
    http://www.withoutmeasure.com
        International Size Acceptance Association monthly online magazine.

Women, Weight, and Power: Feminist Theoretical and Therapeutic Issues. Laura S. Brown (Spring 1975). *Women & Therapy.*

Women En Large: Images of Fat Nudes. Laurie Toby Edison & Debbie Notkin (1994). Books in Focus.

Worth Your Weight: What You Can Do About a Weight Problem. Barbara Altman Bruno (1996). Rutledge Books.
        Clinical social worker and psychotherapist encourages large people to take themselves seriously, as worthy and deserving.

You Count, Calories Don't. Linda Omichinski (1996). Hugs International.
        Healthy living as a journey of self-discovery.

Zaftig: Well Rounded Erotica. Hanne Blank (2001). Cleis Press.

Fat and Fit

Active at Any Size. National Institutes of Health Publication.
    http://win.niddk.nih.gov/publication/active.htm

Excellent source on the specific concerns larger people have when exercising.

Big Moves: Yoga for Chair and Bed. Mara Nesbitt, LMT with Molly Gorger (2001, 2002). Mirage Video Productions.

Don't Weight! Eat Healthy and Get Moving NOW! Kelly Bliss (2001). Xlibris.

> Kelly Bliss' website is the best source for this book: http://www.kellybliss.com.

Empowering Women Through Movement
> Rochelle Rice
> 555 Third Avenue
> New York, NY 10016
> 212–689–4558
> 877–943–7749
> http://www.infitnessinhealth.com/

Fat Friendly Health Professionals
> http://cat-and-dragon.com/stef/fat/ffp.html
> This online list is updated regularly and provides consumer information regarding health care professionals who provide better than average (and sometimes excellent) health care for larger folks.

Feeling Good Fitness
> Jennifer Portnick
> http://www.feelinggoodfitness.com/
> Advocate for "fit and fat" philosophy, speaker, consultant and aerobic instructor.

Fitness with Bliss
> 1–877-KellyBliss
> http://www.kellybliss.com/products/1ml.shtml
> Series of 12 workout videos designed for large and superlarge people.

Great Shape: The First Fitness Guide for Large Women. Pat Lyons & Debby Burgard (2000, 1988). iUniverse.

Health Risks of Weight Loss. Frances M. Berg (1993). *Obesity & Health.*

Just the Weigh You Are: How to Be Fit and Healthy Whatever Your Size. Steven Jonas & Linda Konner (1998). Houghton Mifflin Co., Ltd.
> This book presents a plan for total fitness and healthy living no matter what your size.

Kelly Bliss
> http://kellybliss.com
> Excellent source for exercise and size acceptance resources.

Obtaining Quality Health Care. NAAFA Health Committee Chair Lynn Meletiche, RN, BS.
> 60 minute cassette tape, available through NAAFA bookstore.

Ready Set Go
> http://www.readysetgo.org
> Ontario Physical Health Educator's Association. Promoting healthy family sports.

Real Fitness for Real Women: A Unique Workout Program for the Plus-Size Woman. Rochelle Rice (2001) .Warner Books.

The Big Mama Wellness Project
> PO Box 385
> Monsey, NY 10952
> http://thebigmama.com
> A non-profit organization promoting healthy lifestyles among big women.

Vitality Leader's Kit
> Health Services and Promotion

Health and Welfare Canada
4th Floor, Jeanne Mance Bldg.
Ottawa, Ontario
Canada K1A 1B4
613–957–8331
fax 613–941–2399
Canadian health-centered materials that focus on a fundamental shift to Health At Any Size and prevention of weight and eating problems.

Fat Kids

A Porcupine Named Fluffy. Helen Lester (1986). Houghton Mifflin.

All Shapes and Sizes: Promoting Fitness and Self-Esteem in Your Overweight Child. Teresa Pitman & Miriam Kaufman (1994). Harper Collins.

Am I Fat? Helping Your Children Accept Differences in Body Size. Joanne Ikeda & Priscilla Naworski (1992). ETR Associates.

Are You Too Fat, Ginny? Karin Jasper (1988). Is Five Press.
For young girls, challenges myths about fatness and dieting, offering the healthy alternative of self-acceptance.

Belinda's Bouquet. Leslea Newman (1991). Alyson Publications.
Small book for all ages. When Belinda is teased about her weight, a flower garden shows her the beauty of diversity.

Blubber. Judy Blume (1976). Bantam Doubleday Dell.
Part of the Books for Young Readers series, about a fat girl.

Breaking Size Prejudice
Twila Ortiz
Dept. of FCS/UW CES
University of Wyoming
Dept. 3354, 1000 E. University Ave.

Laramie, WY 82071
307–766–5375
FAX: 307–766–5686
fcs-orders@uwyo.edu
http://www.uwyo.edu/winwyoming/Breaking_Size_Prejudice.
htm
>Promotes respect and size acceptance; 20-minute video developed by youth, includes skits, teacher's packet, activities, grade 6–9.

Child of Mine: Feeding with Love and Good Sense. Ellyn Satter (2000). Bull Publishing.
>Box 208
>Palo Alto, CA 94302
>800–676–2855

Childhood and Adolescent Obesity in America: What's a Parent To Do? Betty Holmes. University of Wyoming Cooperative Extension Publication #B-1066.
>307–766–2115

Children and Teens Afraid to Eat: Helping Youth in Today's Weight-Obsessed World. Frances M. Berg (2001, 1997). Healthy Weight Network.
>402 South 14th St.
>Hettinger, ND 58639
>http://www.healthyweight.net
>>A new approach to dealing with weight and eating in healthier ways.

Energy Expenditure in African American and White Boys and Girls in a 2-y Follow-Up of the Baton Rouge Children's Study. James P. Delany, George A. Bray, David W. Harsha, & Julia Volaufova (2004). *American Journal of Clinical Nutrition.*

Every Body Is Beautiful: Teaching Children about Size Acceptance. Amy Votava (March/April 2004) *Mothering.*

http://www.mothering.com/articles/body_soul/bodywise/
body-beautiful.htm
> Great article about how to teach your kids size acceptance.

Good News for Big Kids
National Association to Advance Fat Acceptance (NAAFA)
PO Box 188620
Sacramento, CA 95818
800–442–1214
916–558–6880
Fax 916–558–6881

If My Child is Overweight, What Should I Do About It? Joanne Ikeda
(1990). Publication # 21455, Cooperative Extension Service.
ANR Communications.
> University of California—Davis
> 800-994-8849
> http://anrcatalog.ucdavis.edu (click on Nutrition & Eating)

Jelly Belly. Robert Kimmel Smith (1982). Bantam Doubleday Dell.
Part of the Books for Young Readers series, about a fat boy.

Kid's Project
Council on Size & Weight Discrimination
Miriam Berg
P.O. Box 305
Mt. Marion, NY 12456
914–679–1209
fax 914–679–1206
> Packet of size acceptance materials. Kids Come in all Sizes
> workshops.

One Fat Summer. Robert Lipsyte (1977). Harper & Row.

Real Kids Come in All Sizes: Ten Essential Lessons to Build Your Child's Body Esteem. Kathy Kater (2004). Broadway Books.

Fat Camp Commandos. Daniel Pinkwater (2001). Scholastic Press. And *Fat Camp Commandos Go West.* Daniel Pinkwater (2003). Scholastic Press.

Stories about fat kids without weight loss moral.

The Pig-Out Blues. Jan Greenberg (1982). Farrar, Straus & Giroux.

Underage and Overweight: America's Childhood Obesity Crisis— and What Families Can Do About It. Frances M. Berg (2004). Hatherleigh Press.

When Girls Feel Fat: Helping Girls Through Adolescence. Sandra Susan Friedman (2000). Firefly Books.

http://www.salal.com

Junk Science

Dispensing With the Truth: The Victims, the Drug Companies, and the Dramatic Story Behind the Battle over Fen-Phen. Alicia Mundy (2001). St. Martin's Press.

Junk Science on the Web: All the Junk That's Fit to Debunk

http://junkscience.com

Drawback: Doesn't really admit to its own agenda even though it is criticizing other agendas. Advantage: Best discussion of reading scientific research found on the web.

National Council Against Health Fraud

http://www.ncahf.org

Has some good information about what to look for in diet scams.

Protecting America's Health: The FDA, Business, and One Hundred Years of Regulation. Philip J. Hilts (2002). Knopf.

Weight Bias among Health Professionals Specializing in Obesity. Marlene B. Schwartz, Heather O'Neal Chambliss, Kelly D. Brownell,

Steven N. Blair, & Charles Billington (2003). *Obesity Research.* http://www.size-acceptance.org/downloads/weight_bias_among.pdf

Media Literacy

About Face
> http://www.about-face.org
> Media literacy organization focused on the impact mass media has on the physical, mental, and emotional well-being of women and girls, and engendering positive body-esteem.

Beginner's Guide to Media Reform
> http://www.freepress.net/guide/
> Good information regarding how media works.

Center for Media Literacy
> http://medialit.org
> 800–226–9494

Disinformation
> http://www.disinfo.com
> 163 Third Avenue, Suite 108
> New York, NY 10003

Just Think Foundation
> http://www.justthink.org
> Information for students, educators and the entertainment industry on promoting media literacy.

Living in the Image Culture: An Introductory Primer for Media Literacy Education. Francis Davis (1992). Center for Media and Values.

Media Awareness Network
> http://www.media-awareness.ca

Media Watch
> http://www.mediawatch.ca
> PO Box 618
> Santa Cruz, CA 95061
> 408–423–6355
>> Website and newsletter dedicated to fighting sexism and violence in media.

Mind on The Media
> http://www.mindonthemedia.org
>> Media watchers dedicated to critical appraisal of body image messages in the media.

Robert McChesney
> http://robertmchesney.com
>> University of Illinois at Urbana-Champaign professor— well-known advocate of free speech and media reform.

Products & Services

Amplestuff
> PO Box 116
> Bearsville, NY 12409
> 914–679–3316
> http://www.amplestuff.com
>> Catalog for large size equipment & other resources for large people.

I'm A Big Gal
> http://www.imabiggal.com

Large Directory
> http://www.largedirectory.com/
>> Online directory for products designed for larger people.

Plus-size Yellow Pages
> http://www.plussizeyellowpages.com/

Best place on the web for larger people to find every kind of resource available for their personal needs.

Size Wise: A Catalog of More Than 1000 Resources for Living with Confidence and Comfort at Any Size. Judy Sullivan (1997). Avon Books.
Resources of all kinds for persons of size; some youth materials.

Stigma and Diversity

A Place at the Table: Memorial to Victims of Fat Phobia and Size Prejudice
http://www.seafattle.org/APATT/apatt.htm

Confessing Excess: Women and the Politics of Body Reduction. Carole Spitzack (1990). State University of New York Press.

Council on Size and Weight Discrimination
Box 305
Mt. Marion NY 12456
914–679–1209
http://www.cswd.org

Full-Figured Women Fight Back: Resistance Grows to Society's Demand for Slim Bodies. Roxanne Brown (March 1990). *Ebony.*

Interpreting Weight: The Social Management of Fatness and Thinness. Jeffery Sobal & Donna Maurer (1999). Aldine de Gruyter.

The Invisible Woman: Confronting Weight Prejudice in America. W. Charisse Goodman (1995). Gurze Books.

Hollywood's Big New Minstrel Show. Melissa Metzler (Winter 2001). *Bitch.*

Nigger: The Strange Career of a Troublesome Word. Randall Kennedy

(2003). Vintage.

Obesity as a Culture-Bound Syndrome. Cheryl Ritenbaugh (1982). *Culture, Medicine and Psychiatry.*

On Being a Fat Black Girl in a Fat-Hating Culture. Margaret K. Bass in *Recovering the Black Female Body: Self-Representations by African American Women,* Michael Bennett & Vanessa D. Dickerson, Eds. (2001). Rutgers University Press.

Our Kind of People. Lawrence Otis Graham (1999). HarperCollins Publishers.

Recent Lawsuits about Fat Discrimination
   http://www.naafa.org/info/legal/coourt.html
      Webpage maintained by NAAFA tracking size discrimination cases in the United States.

Shadow on a Tightrope: Writings by Women on Fat Oppression. Lisa Schoenfielder & Barb Wieser, Eds. (1983). Aunt Lute Books.

Sister Outsider. Audre Lorde, Ed. (1977). The Crossing Press.

Size: The Other Diversity. Veronica Cook-Euell (August 2004). *Mosaics: Society for Human Resource Management Focuses on Workplace Diversity.*
      Excellent article about the costs of fat discrimination in human resources.

Size Matters, Too
   Veronica Cook-Euell
   WCRS FM Radio
   Euell Consulting Group, LLC
   PO Box 8369
   Akron, Ohio 44320–8369
   330–668–6666
   http://www.theeuellconsultinggroup.com/sizematters.asp

Consulting firm and weekly internet radio show dedicated to promoting size acceptance and fighting size discrimination.

Stigma: Notes on the Management of Spoiled Identity. Erving Goffman (1986/1963). Touchstone.

The Construction, Deconstruction, and Reconstruction of Difference. Paula Rothenberg in *Hatred, Bigotry, and Prejudice: Definitions, Causes & Solutions,* Robert M. Baird & Stuart E. Rosenbaum, Eds. (1990). Prometheus Books.

The Forbidden Body: Why Being Fat is Not a Sin. Shelley Bovey (1994). Pandora Press.

The Managed Heart: Commercialization of Human Feeling. Arlie Hochschild (2003/1983). University of California Press.
    Not directly about stigma, but a good examination of how presenting a "self" to others is mediated by the judgments of others.

The Negro Leagues and the Contradictions of Social Darwinism. Alex Ruck & Rob Ruck in *Baseball and Philosophy: Thinking Outside the Batter's Box,* Eric Bronson, Ed. (2004). Open Court Publishing Company.

Tipping the Scales of Justice: Fighting Weight-Based Discrimination. Sondra Solovay (2000). Prometheus Books.
    An attorney fighting discrimination based on size.

Unbearable Weight: Feminism, Western Culture, and the Body. Susan Bordo (1993). University of California Press.

White Racism. Joe R. Feagin & Hernan Vera (1995). Routledge.

White Trash: Race and Class in America. Matt Wray & Annalee Newitz, Ed. (1996) Routledge.

Study of Social Problems

Challenges and Choices: Constructionist Perspectives on Social Problems. Jim Holstein & Gale Miller (2003). Aldine.

Institutional Selves: Troubled Identities in a Postmodern World. James A. Holstein & Jaber F. Gubrium (2000). Oxford University Press.

Social Problems in Everyday Life: Studies of Social Problems Work. Gale Miller & Jim Holstein (1997). JAI Press.

Thinking about Social Problems. An Introduction to Constructive Perspectives. Donileen Loseke (1999). Aldine de Gruyter.

Weighty Issues: Fatness and Thinness as Social Problems. Jeffery Sobal & Donna Maurer (1999). Aldine de Gruyter.

War on Obesity

Rocky Mountain News columnist
Paul Campos, J.D.
http://www.rockymountainnews.com/drmn/columnist/0,1299,DRMN_86_105,00.html
Incredible body of work examining the war on obesity and obesity research.

Tech Central Station columnist
Sandy Szwarc, R.N.
http://www.techcentralstation.com/bioszwarcsandy.html
Incredible body of work examining the war on obesity. obesity research and nutritional research.

The 'War' Against Obesity. Radley Balko (June 25, 2004). Cato Institute.
http://www.cato.org/dailys/06-25-04-2.html

The Cato Institute is a libertarian-funded think tank with a specific agenda of keeping government out of personal lives.

The War on Fat: Is the Size of Your Butt the Government's Business? Jacob Sullum (August/September 2004). *Reason.*
http://www.reason.com/0408/fe.js.the.shtml
Good outline of many of the players in the war on obesity.

Toward Sensitive Treatment of Obese Patients. Syed M Ahmed, Jeanne Parr Lemkau, & Sandra Lee Birt (2002.) *Family Practice Management.*

Weight Loss Surgery

Gastric Surgery for the Severely Obese. National Institutes of Health (December 2001). NIH Publication No. 01–4006.
http://www.niddk.nih.gov/health/nutrit/pubs/gastric/gastricsurgery.htm

I Want to Live: Gastric Bypass Reversal. Dana Hart (2002). Mountain Stars.
http://www.mtnstars.com/

Obesity Surgery Information Center
http://gastricbypass.netfirms.com/
A comprehensive website dedicated to giving full disclosure regarding all forms of weight loss surgery. Strives to provide an informed consent point-of-view rather than advocating a particular decision.

Body Size Calculus

1. See "Theoretical Underpinnings for Women's Health" by McBride & Bride (1981)

2 See Laura Fraser's *Losing It* (1998) for a complete description of the industry dedicated to weight loss.

3. As quoted by Laura Fraser in *Losing It*, p. 224.

Before & After

1. For more information on prevalence, symptoms and consequences of eating disorders, see fact sheet at http://www.anad.org.

2. See Peter N. Stearns' *Fat History* (1997).

3. See Carole Spitzack's *Confessing Excess* (1990).

4. See Laura S. Brown's "Women, Weight, and Power: Feminist Theoretical and Therapeutic Issues" in the Spring 1975 issue of *Women and Therapy*, pages 61–71.

5. For an extensive outline of these practices and how to deal with them, see The Council on Size and Weight Discrimination at http://www.cswd.org.

6. See Paula Rothenberg's "The Construction, Deconstruction, and Reconstruction of Difference" in *Hatred, Bigotry, and Prejudice: Definitions, Causes & Solutions* (1990).

7. See Glenn Gaesser's *Big Fat Lies* for a complete outline of the literature regarding health, activity and weight.

8. See Delany, J. P. *et al.* "Energy Expenditure in African American and White Boys and Girls in a 2-y Follow-Up of the Baton Rouge Children's Study." *American Journal of Clinical Nutrition*, 79 (2004): 268–73.

Looking Good

1. See Melissa Metzler's editorial "Hollywood's Big New Minstrel Show" in the Winter 2001 issue of *Bitch*.

2. See the Critical Psychiatry web site for an outline of some of the current issues with the brain chemistry approach to psychotherapy. See also Peter Breggin's work on Prozac. I am not asserting that antidepressants do not work. I am merely pointing out that the studies currently conducted rarely ask the basic question about the relationship between brain chemistry and emotions or behavior. They are assuming a relationship that is far from proven, but remains profitable to pharmaceutical companies.

3. There are a number of works where Sandra Harding develops her ideas about strong objectivity and standpoint theory. See especially Chapter 8 of *Is Science Multi-Cultural?: Postcolonialisms, Feminisms, and Epistemologies.*

4. See Harding's *Is Science Multicultural?*, p. 144.

5. See page 153-4 of Glassner's *The Culture of Fear.* This quote comes from an entire chapter that deals with a number of "metaphorical illnesses" throughout American history. It is important to keep in mind that critiquing an illness on the basis of its rhetorical purpose within social contexts is not meant to undermine the personal experiences of sufferers. Calling something a metaphorical illness is not the same as calling it "not real." But there is no doubt that a number of people have suffered more because of the stigma and social ostracism that can occur when the social contexts are not examined. In addition to Harding's and Glassner's critiques of the social construction of diseases, I would recommend reading *The Structure of Scientific Resolutions* by Thomas Kuhn, *The Turning Point* by Fritjof Capra, *The Flight to Objectivity* by Susan Bordo and *Ideas and Opinions* by Albert Einstein.

6. See the "Critiques of Obesity Science" in the Resource Appendix.

7. See Alan M. Dershowitz's *The Abuse Excuse: And Other Cop-outs, Sob Stories, and Evasions of Responsibility* for cases of people using "sickness" to redefine "criminality."

8. See Alicia Mundy's *Dispensing with the Truth* for more information regarding the FDA process in approving Redux. Details regarding the class action suits for victims of phen-fen, Redux and Meridia can be found on the website http://www.classactionamerica.com/Current-Cases/Current-cases.asp.

9.   See Laura Fraser's *Losing It*, pages 195–202 for a complete discussion of the Phen-Fen/Redux FDA history.

10.   See *The Obesity Myth* by Paul Campos, especially Chapter 17, for an excellent discussion of the ways in which different players in the obesity game are invested in the notion that fat is deadly.

11.   See "Obesity, Health, and Metabolic Fitness" by Glen Gaesser (*Think Muscle:* http://www.thinkmuscle.com/articles/gaesser/obesity.htm) and "Losing Weight—An Ill-fated Resolution" by Jerome P. Kassirer, MD and Marcia Angell, M.D. (*New England Journal of Medicine*, Editorial, 1 January 1998, also found at http://generous.net/health/nejm.shtml) for discussions of the complexities of body fat and metabolic health.

12.   One of the difficulties in writing about the current climate in the war on fat is that the climate is getting worse by the day. Within in hours of writing that no one was showing before and after pictures of organs, I came across an article about the end of the Time-Warner/ABC Obesity Summit (June 4–5, 2004) that outlined recommendations made by the participants. Among those recommendations is the encouragement of showing organs "damaged by obesity." I'm not exactly sure how one can do this since, unlike the black lungs damaged by the tar found in cigarettes showed to me in sixth grade to discourage me from smoking (something I had already tried by then) and the "stuff-on-the-wall-that-used-to-be-a-human-being" showed to me in eleventh grade to discourage me from drunk driving, I know of no clear effect that obesity has on any particular organ. Still, I do not think that the showing of organs demonstrates a clear concern for the health of fat people. This suggestion smacks of pure sensationalism. If health were the notion, then I'd like to see organs that look better after weight loss. My guess is that it would be easier to present organs that have been damaged after weight loss attempts (heart valves come to mind) than it would be to present organs "damaged by obesity." In the end, it is still about how things look. Claudia Willis, editor-at-large for *Time* and moderator for the Obesity Summit summed up the thinking regarding presentations of this sort to schoolchildren, "the very grossness of it was very powerful."

13.   See NAAFA's web site http://www.naafa.org for the press release.

Building Strength

1.   See http://www.seafattle.org/APATT/VicDD.html for a chronology of various drugs and supplements that have been responsible for killing people in the

name of weight loss, from 1893 to the present.

2. See http://www.seafattle.org/APATT/apattmems.html for a collection of personal stories in memory of those who have died young due to weight loss attempts. The table is not a complete picture, but it is certainly a powerful one.

3. The Center for Science in the Public Interest (CSPI) keeps a database of corporate sponsorship for non-profit and scientific research. The original "million dollar" sponsors of the so-called "federal initiative" included Weight Watchers International, Campbell Soup Company, Heinz Foundation, Time, Kellogg Company, Jenny Craig, and SlimFast Foods Company. Other projects and conferences since the original announcement have had additional sponsorship from the National Cattlemen's Beef Association, Wyeth-Ayerst, Aventis, Dairy Management, Inc., Kellogg Company, SlimFast Foods Company, NatraTaste, Ortho-McNeil, RIVA Market Research, Ross Nutrition, Tanita Corporation of America, Inc., The Robert Wood Johnson Foundation, Ethicon Edno-Surgery, Inc. and Novartis Nutrition. The CSPI does not make a judgment on the inherent conflicts of interest that might or might not be present in these kinds of sponsorships, but has set up the data base in the interest of the public knowing that such relationships exist because they are frequently not part of press releases and public statements.

4. Paul Campos, in *The Obesity Myth*, outlines these claims and demonstrates aptly the problems with these claims. For the moment, I wish to examine the process of these claims rather than their validity.

5. The Cato Institute (admittedly a group with an agenda, and not one that is always friendly to fat people) criticized the handling of the 2001 terrorist attacks by HHS because it misused the USPHS by sending them out to handle acute care during 9/11 attacks in New York, but was not able to put their epidemiologists in charge of the anthrax investigations later that year. Cato sees the fallout from 9/11 being the expansion of federal powers and the reduction of the USPHS. For more information about the USPHS, see their website: http://www.usphs.gov.

6. Since writing this, a public health crisis demonstrating gaps in the public health system has occurred in the form of flu vaccines. In the fall of 2004, a shortage of vaccines was created when one of only two companies making the vaccines had to throw out their stock due to contamination. Media coverage indicated shock at the poorly organized dependency on two foreign companies to protect the American public from epidemics. The flu vaccine shortage is a perfect example of the issues that need to be raised regarding public health in the United States and, unfortunately, may be a hint of more crises to come. So even dis-

eases that fit nicely within the medical model are now affected by a "for profit" medical system and a public health system born from reactivity rather than pro-activity and suffering from "gaps."

7. The dominant notion of western medicine is that human bodies can be studied as a single grouping with a mechanical and universal point of view. This means that the body is simply the sum of its parts and that understanding the parts of a human body tells the medical researcher and physician everything that is needed to identify and cure disease. This paradigm suggests that the properties of cells, organs or systems are more important than the whole body, including subjective experience. In this paradigm, illness and cures are found in the parts of the body. Health is the absence of illness or the return to an absence of illness. Such a notion makes quantification of disease quite simple; however, it tends to miss a lot of information and begs a lot of questions about health and well being. Most medical researchers and physicians give lip service to complexity and diversity, but they do not abandon their models that are based upon simplicity and universality.

8. The 20-hour workweek is widely reported especially among those organizations that promote a simpler lifestyle, but I was unable to find a specific origin of the estimate. I first heard it on a listserv for whole systems thinkers. The number of hours varies between 15 and 30, but 20 is the number I've seen most often. I remain unsure of the validity of the assertion, but I do believe that the general sentiment is true. No one seems to doubt that people work longer hours to maintain their lifestyles in complex industrial societies than in hunter-gatherer societies.

9. Wells admits, however, to making numerous attempts to lose weight, and he has felt some pressure by management to do so. He spoke out publicly about the pressure when Orioles pitcher Steve Bechler died from complications related to weight loss attempts using the herb ephedra.

Bibliography

Ahmed, Syed M., Jeanne Parr Lemkau, and Sandra Lee Birt. "Toward Sensitive Treatment of Obese Patients." *Family Practice Management* 9, no. 1 (2002): 25–31.

Berg, Frances M. *Afraid to Eat: Children and Teens in Weight Crisis.* Hettinger, ND: Healthy Living Institute, 1997.

Bernell, Bonnie. *Bountiful Women: Large Women's Secrets for Living the Life They Desire.* Berkeley, CA: Wildcat Canyon Press, 2000.

Bordo, Susan. *Unbearable Weight: Feminism, Western Culture and the Body.* Berkeley, CA: University of California Press, 1993.

The Boston Women's Health Book Collective. *Our Bodies, Ourselves: A Book by and for Women.* New York: Touchstone, 1992.

Brown, Laura S. "Women, Weight, and Power: Feminist Theoretical and Therapeutic Issues." *Women and Therapy,* Spring (1975): 61–71.

Campos, Paul. *The Obesity Myth.* New York: Gotham Books, 2004

Charmez, Kathy. *Good Days, Bad Days: The Self in Chronic Illness and Time.* New Brunswick, NJ: Rutgers University Press, 1991.

Chernin, Kim. *The Obsession Reflections on the Tyranny of Slenderness.* New York: HarperPerennial, 1994.

Delany, James P., Bray, George A., Harsha, David W., & Volaufova, Julia. "Energy Expenditure in African American and White Boys and Girls in a 2-y Follow-up of the Baton Rouge Children's Study." *American Journal of Clinical Nutrition* 79 (2004): 268–73.

Feagin, Joe R. and Hernan Vera. *White Racism.* New York: Routledge, 1995.

Fraser, Laura. *Losing It: False Hopes and Fat Profits in the Diet Industry.* New York: Plume Books, 1998.

Freedman, Rita. *Beauty Bound.* Lexington, MA: Lexington Books, 1986.

Gaesser, Glenn A. *Big Fat Lies: The Truth About Your Weight and Your Health.* 1st ed., New York: Fawcett Columbine, 1996.

Gaesser, Glenn A. "Is It Necessary to be Thin to be Healthy?" *The Harvard Review,* 4.2 (2003): 40–47.

Glassner, Barry. *Culture of Fear.* New York: Basic Books, 2000.

Goffman, Erving. *Stigma : Notes on the Management of Spoiled Identity.* New York: Touchstone, 1986(1963).

Graham, Lawrence Otis. *Our Kind of People.* 1st ed., New York: HarperCollins Publishers, 1999.

Harding, Sandra. *Is Science Multi-Cultural?: Postcolonialisms, Feminisms, and Epistemologies.* Bloomington, IN: Indiana University Press, 1998.

Hillman, James. *The Soul's Code.* New York: Warner Books, 1996.

Kilbourne, Jean. *Can't Buy My Love: How Advertising Changes the Way We Think and Feel.* New York: Touchstone, 2000.

Lappe, Frances Moore. *Diet for a Small Planet.* New York: Ballantine Books, 1991.

Lerner, Harriet. *The Dance of Anger: A Woman's Guide to Changing the Patterns of Intimate Relationships.* New York: Perennial Library, 1985.

Lorde, Audre. "The Transformation of Silence into Language and Action." *Sister Outsider.* Ed. Audre Lorde. Freedom, CA: The Crossing Press, 1977: 40–44.

Lorde, Audre. "The Uses of Anger: Women Responding to Racism." *Sister Outsider.* Ed. Audre Lorde. Freedom, CA: The Crossing Press, 1981: 124–33.

Lorde, Audre. "Uses of the Erotic: The Erotic As Power." *Sister Outsider*. Ed. Audre Lorde. Freedom, CA: The Crossing Press, 1978: 53–59.

Loseke, Donileen. *Thinking about Social Problems*. New York: Aldine de Gruyter, 1999.

Manheim, Camryn. *Wake Up, I'm Fat!* New York: Broadway Books, 1999.

McBride, A. B. and W. L. McBride. "Theoretical Underpinnings for Women's Health." *Women & Health* (1981): 6:37–55.

Metzler, Melissa. "Hollywood's Big New Minstrel Show." *Bitch*, Winter (2001).

National Task Force on the Prevention and Treatment of Obesity. "Medical Care for Obese Patients: Advice for Health Care Professionals." *American Family Physician* 65 (2002): 81–88.

Orbach, Susan. *Fat is A Feminist Issue*. New York: Berkley, 1979.

Ritenbaugh, Cheryl. "Obesity as a culture-bound syndrome." *Culture, Medicine and Psychiatry*, 6 (1982): 347–59.

Roth, Geneen. *Feeding the Hungry Heart*. Indianapolis, NY: Bobbs-Merrill Co. Inc., 1982.

Rothenberg, Paula. "The Construction, Deconstruction, and Reconstruction of Difference." *Hatred, Bigotry, and Prejudice: Definitions, Causes & Solutions*. Robert M. Baird & Stuart E. Rosenbaum, Eds. Amherst, NY: Prometheus Books, 1990: 107–24.

Ruck, Alex and Rob Ruck. "The Negro Leagues and the Contradictions of Social Darwinism." *Baseball and Philosophy: Thinking Outside the Batter's Box*. Ed. Eric Bronson. Peru, IL: Open Court Publishing Company, 2004.

Schor, Juliet B. *The Overspent American*. New York: Basic Books, 1998.

Seid, Roberta P. *Never Too Thin: Why Women Are at War With Their Bodies*. New York: Prentice Hall, 1991.

Spitzack, Carole. *Confessing Excess: Women and the Politics of Body Reduction*. Albany, NY: State University of New York Press, 1990.

Stearns, Peter N. *Fat History: Bodies and Beauty in the Modern West*. New York University Press, 1997.

Thomas, Pattie. "An Interview with Paul Campos." *Big Fat Blog.* 2004. http://www.bigfatblog.com/columnists/archives/001240.php.

Wann, Marilyn. *FAT!SO?: Because You Don't Have to Apologize for Your Size!* Berkeley, CA: Ten Speed Press, 1998.

Weiss, Michael. *The Clustering of America.* New York: Harpercollins, 1988.

Wolf, Naomi. *The Beauty Myth: How Images of Beauty Are Used Against Women.* New York: William Morrow and Company, Inc., 1991.

— Index

ENJOY · ENLARGE · ENLIGHTEN · ENLIVEN
your Self

To find other inspirational and empowering books
published by Pearlsong Press:

go to: www.pearlsong.com
call: 1-866-4-A-PEARL
or write to   Pearlsong Press
                  P.O. Box 58065
                  Nashville, TN 37205

For news about Pearlsong Press books, authors and promotions,
see our blog at www.pearlsongpress.com
or subscribe to *The Pearlsong Letter* at
www.pearlsong.com/subscribe.htm.

Printed in the United States
50007LVS00003B/29

9 781597 190022

UN. General Assembly (60th sess.: 2005-2006). *2005 World Summit Outcome Resolution*. Vol. 60. New York: UN, 2005.

UNDP. *Human Development Report 2007/2008: Human Development and Climate Change*. Palgrave Macmillan, 2008. *http://hdr. undp.org/en/reports/global/hdr2007-2008/*.

UNICEF. *The 'Rights' Start to Life: A statistical analysis of birth registration*. UNICEF, February 2005. *http://www.unicef.org/ publications/files/BirthReg10a_rev.pdf*.

United Nations. *Housing and Property Restitution in the Context of the Return of Refugees and Internally Displaced Persons: Final Report of the Special Rapporteur, Paulo Sérgio Pinheiro: Principles on Housing and Property Restitution for Refugees and Displaced Persons*. E/CN.4/SUB.2/2005/17. Geneva: UN. *http://daccessdds.un.org/doc/UNDOC/GEN/G05/146/95/PDF/ G0514695.pdf?OpenElement*.

United Nations. *Interim Report of the Special Representative of the Secretary-General on the Issue of Human Rights and Transnational Corporations and Other Business Enterprises*. Geneva: UN.

United Nations. *The Millennium Development Goals Report 2007*. United Nations, 2007.

United Nations. *The Universal Declaration of Human Rights*. New York: King Typographic Service Corp, 1949. *http://www.unhchr.ch/ udhr/lang/eng.pdf*.

USAID. *Removing Barriers to Formalization: The Case for Reform and Emerging Best Practice*. USAID, 2005. *http://www.oecd.org/ dataoecd/36/27/38452590.pdf*.

World Bank. *Economic Growth in the 1990s: Learning from a Decade of Reform*. Washington, D.C: World Bank, 2005.

World Bank. 'IDA - 2005 IDA Resource Allocation Index (IRAI).' *http://go.worldbank.org/MY944F3BN0*.

World Bank. *Water Resources Sector Strategy: Strategic Directions for World Bank Engagement*. World Bank Publications, 2004.

World Bank. *World Development Indicators 2007*. World Bank. *http://siteresources.worldbank.org/DATASTATISTICS/Resources/ WDI07frontmatter.pdf*.

World Bank. *World Development Report 2005: A Better Investment Climate for Everyone*. World Bank Publications, 2004. *http://go. worldbank.org/WVDAOSZJ20*.

World Bank. *World Development Report 2006: Equity and Development*. World Bank; Palgrave [distributor], 2006. *http://go.worldbank. org/UWYLBR43C0*.

WIPO 2005 'Intellectual Property and Traditional Knowledge,' Booklet No 2. Publication No. 920(E). *http://www.wipo.int/ freepublications/en/tk/920/wipo_pub_920.pdf*

World Resource Institute, ed. *World Resources 2005 – The Wealth of the Poor: Managing ecosystems to fight poverty*, 2005. *http:// archive.wri.org/publication_detail.cfm?pubid=4073*.

Yeng, José and S. Cartier van Dissel. 'Improving access of small local contractors to public procurement – The experience of Andean Countries,' *ASIST Bulletin* No. 18, September 2004, International Labour Organisation.